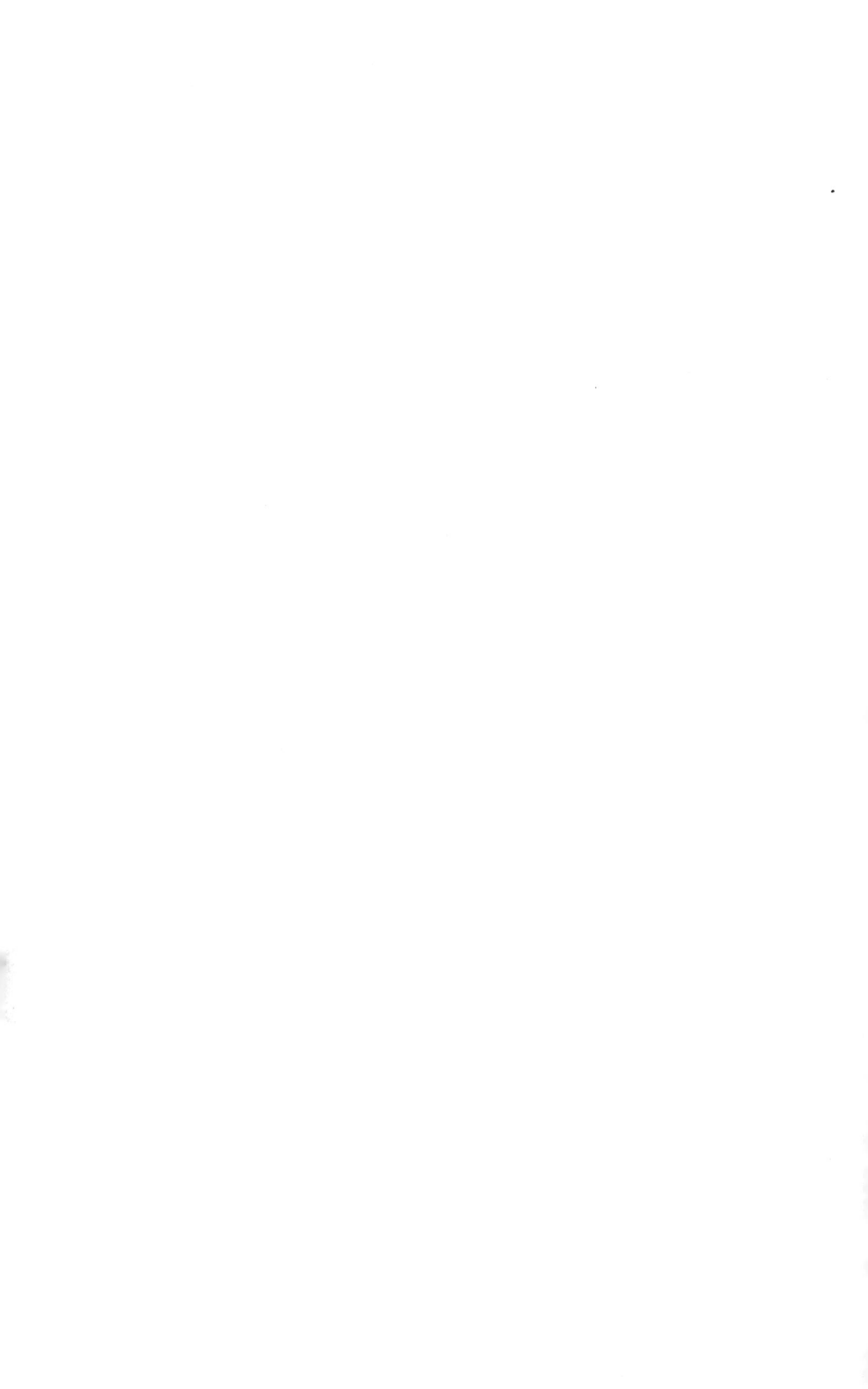

THE QUALITY REVOLUTI
A Primer for Purcha

by
M. Dani
Michael C

THE QUALITY REVOLUTION AND HEALTH CARE
A Primer for Purchasers and Providers

by
M. Daniel Sloan
Michael Chmel, MD

THE QUALITY REVOLUTION AND HEALTH CARE
A Primer for Purchasers and Providers

by
M. Daniel Sloan
Michael Chmel, MD

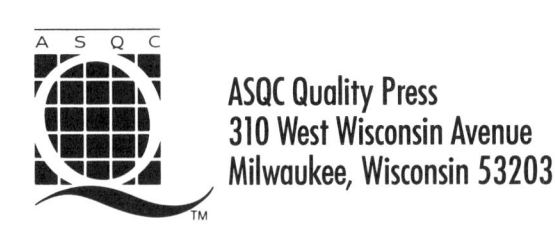

ASQC Quality Press
310 West Wisconsin Avenue
Milwaukee, Wisconsin 53203

THE QUALITY REVOLUTION AND HEALTH CARE
A Primer for Purchasers and Providers

M. Daniel Sloan
Michael Chmel, MD

Library of Congress Cataloging-in-Publication Data

Sloan, M. Daniel.
   The quality revolution and health care : a primer for purchasers and providers / M. Daniel Sloan, Michael Chmel.
     p. cm.
   Includes bibliographical references.
   ISBN 0-87389-098-1
   1. Medical care — Quality control — Statistical methods.
2. Medical care — Cost control. I. Chmel, Michael. II. Title.
RA3 99.A3S56 1991
362.1'068'5 -- dc20   90-25575
                                                                                             CIP

Copyright © 1991 by ASQC Quality Press
All rights reserved. No part of this book may be reproduced in any form or by any means, electronic, mechanical, photocopying, recording, or otherwise, without the prior permission of the publisher.

10987654321

ISBN 0-87389-098-1

Acquisitions Editor: Jeanine L. Lau
Production Editor: Tammy Griffin
Set in Century Schoolbook by DanTon Typographers. Cover design by Artistic License.
Printed and bound by Port City Press.

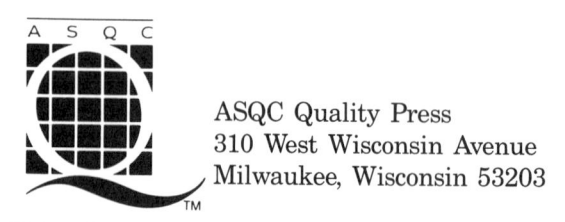

ASQC Quality Press
310 West Wisconsin Avenue
Milwaukee, Wisconsin 53203

Printed in the United States of America

For Lynne and Austin, Jeanie and Briana

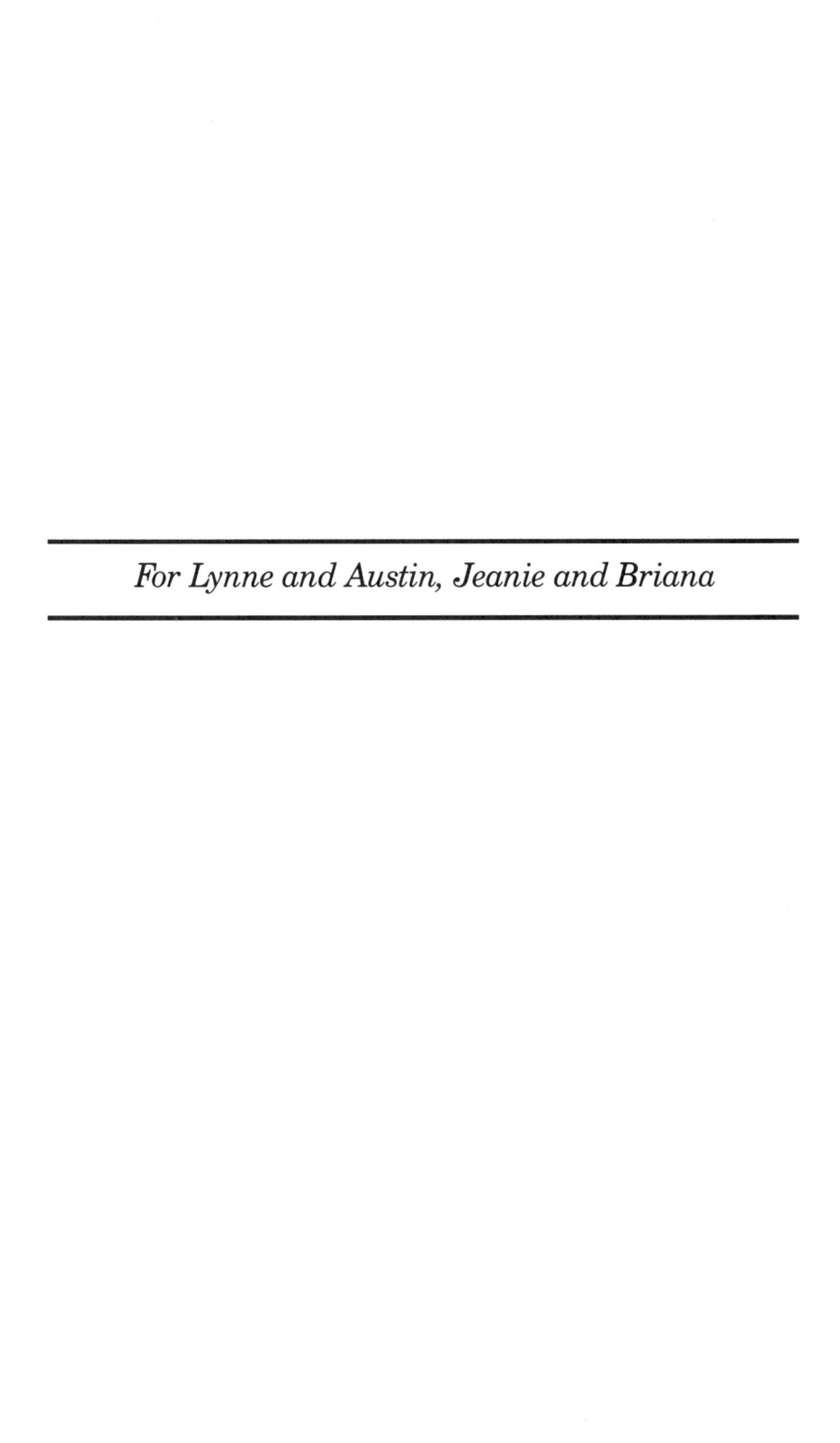

Contents

Acknowledgments .... **ix**

Prologue .... **xi**

Chapter 1
On Call—March 1990 1

Chapter 2
Health Care Chaos 5
   Misbehavior 7
   Psychological Distress 10
   End of Life Expenses 11
   Systemic Cynicism 12

Chapter 3
The Quality Approach 19

Chapter 4
Cast of Characters 35
   Patient 36
   Physician 37
   Administrator 40

Chapter 5
Twenty-Two Hours and 45 Minutes—March 1990 43
   Act One 43
   Act Two 59

Chapter 6
World Class Health Care 73
   New Knowledge and the Scientific Revolution 74
      C. I. Lewis, Outline of a Theory of Knowledge 75
      W. A. Shewhart, Three Components of Knowledge 77
   The World Class Health Care Process 84
   Hospitalization As a Teachable Moment 91
   Integrated Treatment 92
      Plan, Do, Check, Act 93
      Medical Cost Offset Effect 96
      Education 101
      Process Quality Control 104

Chapter 7
Quality Initiatives **115**
   Individual Initiative 116
   Family Initiative 119
   Employer Initiative 120
   Congressional Initiative 131

Epilogue 2010 .... **135**

Sources and Recommended Reading **137**

Appendix A
   Sample Certification Program **149**

Appendix B
   World Class Health Care versus Medical Tradition:
   Case Studies **169**

Index **189**

Acknowledgments

Both authors extend their thanks to Dr. John Striebel, Alma Williams, Mardy Fones, Jeanine Lau, Gloria and Steve Eller. Dr. Striebel made substantive contributions to the development of World Class Health Care theory and the descriptions of behavioral medicine theory contained in *The Quality Revolution and Health Care*. Mrs. Williams provided superior market research assistance. Mardy and Jeanine gave editorial direction. Gloria and Steve gave gifts of encouragement, graphic design, and photography.

ASQC played an instrumental role in the evolution and final form of this book.

Carter Center Study conclusions from *Closing the Gap* have been referenced with permission of the Oxford University Press and the *Journal of Preventive Medicine*.

Passages and illustrations from Walter Shewhart's *Economic Control of Quality of Manufactured Product* and *Statistical Method from the Viewpoint of Quality Control* are reprinted with permission of ASQC.

Passages from C.I. Lewis' *Mind and the World Order* are used with permission of Andrew Lewis.

Illustrations adapted from J.M. Juran's *Juran's Quality Control Handbook, Fourth Edition* are used with permission of McGraw-Hill Book Company.

Brief passages from Albert Einstein's *Relativity* are reprinted with permission of Crown Publishers Inc.

Steve deShazer's central map of Brief Therapy is reproduced with permission of W.W. Norton & Company.

The Michigan Alcohol Screening Test is reprinted with permission of M.L. Selzer MD.

A portion of the Beck Depression Inventory is reproduced with permission of the Psychological Corporation, San Antonio, Texas.

Costs of Quality illustrations have been adapted from H. James Harrington's *Poor Quality Costs* with permission of ASQC.

Prologue

Our aim is to help transform health care into a quality industry. Prevention, accurate diagnosis, and treatment plans which mandate teamwork can save millions of lives. A health care system, radically altered through the skillful application of process quality control, can save our nation billions of dollars a year in health care costs.

We wrote this book in two voices. One is for the heart. One is for the head. We crafted our stories so readers could feel the heartache that is our current health care system. We framed decision dilemmas to heighten awareness. We modeled our vision of a healthy future to sharpen perception. Health care purchasers—individuals, families, industry, and government—can claim this future whenever they wish.

If you are certain already that our nation's health care expenditures can and ought to be dramatically reduced, this book should strengthen your conviction. High quality health care and affordable prices are not mutually exclusive; they depend on one another.

Those of us who rely on the hospital industry for our livelihood live with an uncomfortable paradox. We work to restore health, knowing a healthy population would impose an enormous change on our lifestyles. Change could produce a quantum advance in medical science. It could present a singular opportunity for medical scientists, behavioral scientists, and educators. It is an opportunity which rivals the time when, one by one, cartographers discovered our world was round.

Change could also sidetrack careers. Preventing illness, producing rapid recoveries, and preventing relapses would cut billions of dollars from health care expenditures and subsequently reduce our annual collective paycheck. We might lose our jobs.

So our industry too often struts a health care attitude championed by medical tradition. Victor Fuchs, MD, summarized it in his book, *Who Shall Live?**

> For the health professional, the "optimum" level (of health) is the highest level technically attainable regardless of the cost of reaching it.

This mind set is disturbing. It suggests people are best cared for with the apparatus of technology. It overlooks the importance of prevention, accurate diagnosis, cost-effective treatment, and teamwork. It ignores statistical method from the viewpoint of quality control. It is positively cavalier in its approach to expense.

Medical technology is a tool. It is not the central element of quality health care. Brainpower is. If brain work is done well by the patient and the rest of the treatment team, cherished technology can mostly be left on the shelf.

---

*Fuchs VR: *Who Shall Live? Health, Economics and Social Change.* New York: Basic Books, Inc., 1974, p. 19.

Health care expenses must be controlled. As our population ages, the sheer numbers of exponentially expanding need will bankrupt our present payment system.

We chose to use melodrama for a serious purpose. It is appropriate because an honestly portrayed hospital routine is melodrama. We must never allow its serial character to numb us into complacency. This absurd theater of life, death, and treatment is the reason we must restructure our health care system.

Federal and state governments are trying to alter our health care system by restricting access to care. They are using cost containment with mass inspection strategies which focus almost entirely on hospital treatment outcomes. The first approach is an insult to every educated mind in America. It invites an epidemic of illness. It courts a revolution by the poor and underprivileged of our nation.

The mass inspection approach to quality control became obsolete during the 1920s when Walter A. Shewhart, a statistician who worked for Bell Telephone Laboratories, introduced the mathematical theories of statistical process control. The mass inspection of outcomes is a known exercise in futility. It results in tampering. Tampering adds complexity to the system and complexity adds expense. Legislative complexity will neither change our health care system nor save us any money.

Individuals and industry are experimenting with their own initiatives to improve the quality of care while reducing health care costs. So are many medical centers. Their efforts are consumerism at its finest. The chance that individuals, employers, and industry will discover high quality health care as the best way to reduce health care costs is quite good. Hence this book.

Health care consumers (individuals, corporate board members, CEOs, human resource managers, benefit plan administrators, and families) are painfully aware of the inexcusable expense of health care. An increasing number of health care providers are joining this group. We share a growing conviction that health care purchases no longer represent good value.

Use the information in this book and the statistical tools of process quality control; the power of your health care purchasing decisions can cause swift improvements in the quality of health care. Collectively we can effect dramatic reductions in the costs of care by insisting on World Class Health Care.

We changed names and invented places but our fiction is based on fact. Together we can choose to make them facts of history instead of the facts of life.

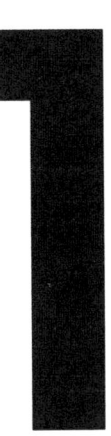

ON CALL—MARCH 1990

The phone rang at 12:05 a.m. Middle-of-the-night phone calls mean trouble.

"Hello," I grouched.

"Roy needs help. Helen can't wake him up!," Roy's daughter-in-law panicked.

"Are you serious?" Of course she was serious. "We're on our way."

I hung up, said, "Roy's down," and watched my wife, Sarah, grab a nightshirt and run out of the bedroom.

Roy had suffered three heart attacks since 1965. He was resilient...and smart. He didn't smoke. He didn't drink. He worked hard around the yard.

All the lights were on in Helen and Roy's home. We ran into their kitchen without knocking. Helen was spinning around in a circle, hands to her cheeks. "He's gone! He's gone! He's gone!"

I thought about how the look on her face begged a photo and how strange it was to think that now.

"Where did you come from?" She was confused.

"Where's Roy?" we asked.

"He's in the bedroom," she answered. "How did you get here?" We ran to the bedroom. Roy's face was blue and gray, and he was on his back. "Call the ambulance!" Sarah ordered. I ran back into the kitchen.

Helen was spinning. "Oh, my God. He's gone. He's gone. He's gone. Oh, my God!"

"Helen! Where's the phone? Where's the phone?" I was impatient. I'll never have a rotary dial phone in my house again. Good thing I run the hospital. If I didn't, I'd probably still be looking for the hospital's number in the phone book instead of waiting for this contraption to ring up Medic 1.

I'll vote twice for the 911 tax levy in the next election.

The telephone rang and rang and rang. I can't believe I laid off that second operator.

"Hello. County Hospital. Can I help you?"

"Yes, you can. Get me the ER. We've got a heart attack here."

The phone transfer took time. Time. Time.

"ER."

"This is David. Our neighbor is down, and we need an ambulance. Quick."

"Who?"

"David Solomon. You know, the administrator. Your boss." I was losing my temper.

"Sorry," she apologized. "Where are you?" Good question.

"I don't know. I don't know my neighbor's address. Jim knows where I live. Just tell him to take the ambulance to my house and tell him to run across the back yard."

"Wait!" the night clerk jumped. "Don't hang up. Find the address. We'll dispatch Medic 1."

"OK. OK."

I looked for Helen. She was gone. Where in the hell could she have gone at a time like this?

"Helen! What's your address?" I demanded. "I don't know where we are. I've got to tell the ambulance where to come."

"856 Bennett."

"856 Bennett. Look, I think we've got to start CPR on Roy," I said. "Have you got the address?"

"Yes. I'll radio it. They're on their way."

"Help me get Roy out of bed," Sarah yelled. Roy hit the floor with a dead heavy thump.

"Are we going to do CPR?"

"Yeah. What do you think?" Sarah asked. "Come on, Roy, Hold on. We're here." She gave me the orders. "You do the chest compressions. I'll work with the airway."

My mind raced. I tried to remember my CPR class. I felt for Roy's xiphoid process.

"One." Twelve ribs crunched in Roy's 70-year-old chest.

"Keep going," Sarah ordered. "Don't stop!"

I began my count again. "One, two, three, four, five."

Sarah blew in air. Roy threw up. Sarah wiped his vomit from her mouth.

It was revolting, but it had to be done.

"One, two, three, four. One, two, three, four, five." A broken rib cage moves easily.

Sarah was telling Roy what to do. Why not? It couldn't hurt. "Breathe, Roy, breathe." She spurred him on. "Wake up. Breathe, Roy, breathe," she repeated. "You'll be fine."

"One, two, three, four, five. His fingers are pink!"

"Hold the compressions." Sarah felt for a pulse. "You've got a heartbeat."

"Let me feel." I cheered, "Helen, he's breathing! Hey! We've got a heartbeat! He's going to make it." It was a premature prognosis, but I was certain.

Two minutes later, three minutes since I'd hung up on the switchboard, the ambulance arrived. Fire department volunteers and paramedics had all the gear they needed—$155,000 on a Ford chassis. I was shaking.

A few minutes later I was home and back in bed with Sarah. There was no way I could sleep. Many things I had taken for granted had just been ripped away from my reality; "what ifs" raced through my mind.

What if I hadn't known how to do CPR?

What if I hadn't known the hospital phone number?

What if there had been no hospital to call?

What if I were Roy?

What if my wife. . .?

What if my son. . .?

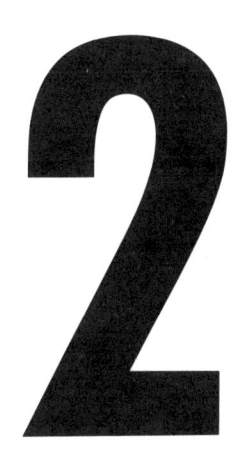

HEALTH CARE CHAOS

Routine life maintains an illusion of security. The specter of Barney Clark's* ghost hovers well beyond the borders of our personal lives as we bankroll a schizophrenic health care system. We spend more than 11 percent of our gross national product—more than $500 billion a year, more than $1.3 billion a day—on health care.

In 1984, Emory University's Carter Center drafted a plan to improve our nation's health care.[1] The published report, *Closing the Gap, The Burden of Unnecessary Illness,* clearly identifies the 14 problems responsible for 80 percent of our direct personal health care costs and 75 percent of hospital care days. They are:

1. Alcoholism
2. Arthritis
3. Cancer
4. Cardiovascular Disease
5. Dental Disease
6. Depression
7. Diabetes
8. Digestive Disease
9. Drug Abuse
10. Homicide/Suicide
11. Infant Mortality
12. Infectious Disease
13. Respiratory Disease
14. Unintended Injuries

---

*Barney Clark received the first Jarvic mechanical heart transplant.

The Carter Center's data summary is a textbook example of the 80/20 rule known in twentieth century quality improvement literature as the Pareto principle.

The Pareto principle was named for a nineteenth century Italian economist, Vilfredo Pareto, who determined that a large amount of his country's wealth was held by a small number of the population.[2] The principle is used to rank order and summarize the primary causes of an observed occurrence. It sorts out the vital few causes from the trivial many.

The Pareto principle can and should be used to simplify any complex decision-making process including health care delivery systems. The Pareto chart (Figure 2.1) is one of the essential statistical tools used by the international quality improvement philosophy.

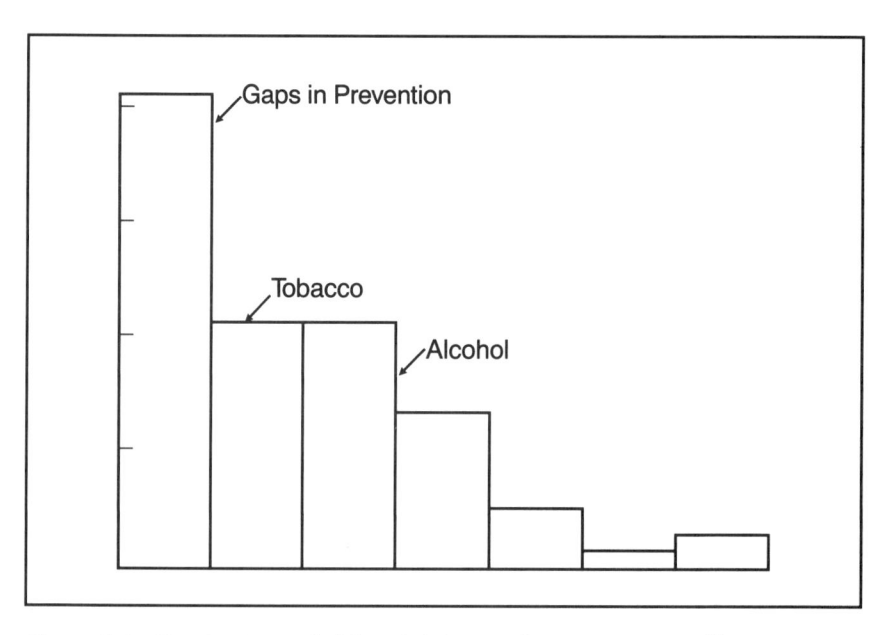

Figure 2.1 Pareto chart: vital few risk factors for unnecessary illness. *(Carter Center Study,*[1] *1987)*

Graphically presented numeric data change the perception of the people who are working on the issue at hand. Statistical pictures unleash the knowledge experts store in their intuition. An apparently overwhelming task broken down into its parts becomes a series of achievable projects.

When the Carter Center further stratified its data, three vital risk factors, vital causes for the 14 problems surfaced. Gaps in primary prevention services are culprits in 12. Primary prevention includes inoculations, education, and health screening. It also includes good personal health habits. Tobacco stands accused in eight. Alcohol abuse is on the docket for eight.

The other causes the Carter Center researchers identified, such as the socioeconomics of poverty, improper nutrition, handguns, and lack of exercise, relative to the three root causes, represent the "trivial" many. None of these risk factors is trivial, but their collective impact on the total problem of unnecessary illness is comparatively small.

The lack of prevention services is a result of our health care system's structure. Tobacco, alcohol, and drug abuse are examples of misbehavior. Misbehavior and health care system structure contribute to health care chaos. In all, four obstacles block our nation's path to quality health care: misbehavior, psychological distress, end of life expenses, and systemic cynicism.

I. Misbehavior

Major illness is rarely a chance occurrence. Catastrophic disease barely surprises. Disease is predictable when people choose to do without sleep, exercise, and a well-balanced diet. Forecasting is further simplified by adding tobacco, mental health problems, alcohol abuse, or drug misuse to the equation. To be sure, genetics predispose each of us to a probable future. How we behave seals our fate.

1. Cardiovascular Disease

Heart disease and vascular disease cause more than half of all deaths in the United States.[1]

- Smoking is responsible for 17 percent of all cardiovascular deaths.[1]
- A diet high in saturated fat contributes to high blood cholesterol. High blood cholesterol is a major risk factor for coronary heart disease and lowering blood cholesterol levels affords significant protection against heart disease.[1,3]

2. Cancer

Bladder cancer, pancreatic cancer, laryngeal cancer, and lung cancer share a common risk factor—smoking.

- Tobacco is the single leading cause of premature death in the United States.[1,4]
- Alcohol misuse and abuse and a high-fat diet are important cancer risk factors.[1]

3. Accidents—Unintended Injuries

Alcohol misuse and other drug abuse are major causes of accidental injuries, especially severe and fatal injuries.

- Alcohol abuse is the second leading cause of premature deaths. Motor vehicle injuries and other unintentional injuries account for two thirds of these deaths.[1,4]
- In a landmark emergency room study, a breathalyzer detected alcohol in 22 percent of home injuries, 16 percent of occupational injuries, and 30 percent of motor vehicle injuries.[1,5]
- Half of all motor vehicle fatalities have a high blood alcohol concentration.[1,6]
- Use of combined lap and shoulder belt reduces the likelihood of death or serious injury by about 50 percent.[1,6]
- Accidental illnesses caused by epidemic cocaine abuse arrive at emergency rooms around the country every day. Cocaine intoxication causes seizures, cardiac arrhythmias, respiratory arrests, and virtually any psychiatric symptom.[7]

4. Cirrhosis

Alcohol abuse is the primary cause of cirrhosis.

- Illnesses directly attributable to alcohol misuse include alcohol psychosis, alcohol polyneuropathy, alcoholic cardiomyopathy, alcoholic gastritis, alcohol dependence syndrome, and acute alcohol toxicity.
- Related illnesses include pneumonia, tuberculosis, and a host of other disorders generalized as alcohol-related debilitation.
- Researchers at the Johns Hopkins University School of Medicine concluded in 1989 that although alcohol dependence or abuse rarely appears as a primary diagnosis, alcoholism is prevalent, on average, in approximately 25 percent of the patients admitted to their hospital.[8]

5. Homicide and Suicide

Violence is a complex problem with many causes. It is rampant in our society.

- In 1980 suicide, homicide, and aggravated assault accounted for more than 50,000 deaths, 1.8 million hospital days, and $754 million in health care costs.[1]
- Of all homicides occurring in 1980, 45 percent were committed by persons known to the victim and nearly a third of those were committed by family members.[1]

- Alcohol misuse and drug abuse are associated with suicide and all types of homicide except child murder.[1]

Why do we repeat behaviors which inevitably lead to illness and premature death? Because they are integral parts of our lifestyle. Familiarity is so gratifying it habituates behavior. Habitual behavior resembles addiction. Over time, addiction rewards even as it leads to sickness.

Lifestyle rewards come easy and they are powerful. Equally satisfying rewards can be gained through endeavor. Love, power, prestige, and recognition motivate and shape behavior. So do money and possessions. Earning rewards is hard work. Getting something for nothing is an opportunity few people pass up. Compulsive gambling will be evident whenever a system of chance rewards exists and people can reasonably expect to get something for nothing.

When we get sick, we get more than our money's worth back in insurance payouts. A single hospital claim can earn an individual more cash benefits than several years, and in many cases, a lifetime, of labor. Convoluted thinking has led some of us to conclude that medical benefits paid are a reward. Similar thinking gave birth to a proliferation of lotteries during the 1980s.

Health care and lotteries are two games people can play for a few dollars and expect to win $50,000, $100,000, or even $1 million. Winners are announced regularly. Everyone knows someone who has won something. Losers are hidden from public view. Heavy losers are too ashamed to expose their staggering gaming expenses.

Our nation's health care and lottery systems differ in a significant way. Lotteries have standardized rules and players must pay each time they play. Health care prizes are won on request.

Medicare and Medicaid established everyone's right to win. It taxes the mind when one realizes these monuments to generosity require more of an investment than millions of people are willing to make. Apparently, the perceived value of today's medical care is not worth the asking price, the price is beyond their means, or people think they might get something for nothing.

According to a 1989 report from American Agenda, Inc.,[9] more than 37 million Americans do not have health insurance. The number of uninsured people is rapidly expanding because health care bills are often excused.

The size of an average hospital bill guarantees sympathy for any person who cannot afford to pay. One-hundred-dollar-per-minute emergency room charges, $1,000-per-quarter-hour operating room prices, and $2,000-per-dose medications stretch the limits of credibility.

Our health care payment system's oddball structure may keep entitlement program prizes disguised forever. Patients frequently feel as though they have lost something even as they claim their winnings. Sometimes they feel slighted, empty, and left in the dark. The rewards we give health care providers are a different story.

Providers are paid exceedingly well to treat disease. If the initial treatment fails to sustain a recovery, higher payments are made for the second treatment. Heroic third and fourth attempts raise the stakes again.

Preventing the first, second, third, or fourth treatment carries a stiff penalty: nonpayment. As long as the penalty remains, many health care industry professionals will understandably argue in favor of treatment.

II. Psychological Distress

Major depression costs our nation more than $16 billion annually.[10] Psychological distress complicates all medical and surgical problems. Anxiety is an expected response to a serious illness.[11] Twelve to 32 percent of medically ill people suffer from depression.[12]

Few medical or surgical patients receive appropriate psychotherapeutic support. Medical and surgical interventions are assumed to be powerful enough to rebuild a patient's health, confidence, and self-esteem. No one expects a patient to perform his or her own surgery. Yet everyone expects the patient to regain a psychological balance independent of expert assistance.

This is an obsolete approach. It exemplifies our culture's overt discrimination against psychological disease. Psychiatric hospitals were originally founded for the same reason as Jewish Hospitals and Catholic Hospitals; undesirables were segregated. Social outcasts who asked for help were refused in their time of need. Our culture denies, minimizes, and consistently ignores the compelling need for routine psychological support.

Health problems are diagnosed by collecting and analyzing facts. The health care scientist has an obligation to collect germane data. Since psychological distress is a probable root cause of an infinite number of medical problems, a behavioral science evaluation performed by a qualified professional is essential to every diagnostic workup. Any diagnosis made without appropriate psychological and lifestyle assessments must be judged to be narrow and always incomplete. Incomplete, and on occasion meaningless, diagnostic protocols result in vast, unknown, and unknowable numbers of misdirected treatments.

Quill[13] wrote about this dilemma in an issue of the *Journal of the American Medical Association*:

> Highly skilled physicians repeatedly fail to recognize patients with somatization disorders...they are better trained to rule out the unusual than to rule in the most probable diagnosis...when forced to confront the psychosocial aspects of illness, we (physicians) enter an area where we often have little inclination to go, much less special training or expertise.

Somatization is the proper word for a psychological or psychosocial illness which masquerades as a physical or organic problem. The preferred description, "It's all in your head," bangs the gong of ignorance.

An abbreviated list of somatization diagnostic criteria includes: difficulty in swallowing, loss of voice, deafness, double vision, blurred vision, seizures and convulsions, paralysis or muscle weakness, abdominal pain, nausea, painful menstruation, pain in the back, joints, and extremities, palpitations, chest pain, and dizziness.

Somatization presents like the real thing because it is the real thing. It has an absolutely infinite capacity to deceive. The destructive thoughts and the emotions which cause these illnesses must first be brought into control if the secondary medical problems are to be resolved.

Brutal consequences await patients who are uninformed about the influence of psychological distress. At best, they may be penalized with a never-ending series of useless tests and treatments. Often, they are admitted to the intensive care units of our most expensive medical centers.

III. End of Life Expenses

People live. People die. Life is arbitrary. Life is capricious. No amount of money will change those facts of existence. Despite the facts, last moments are precious.

We will spend our entire life's savings, our family's nest egg, and our government's treasury to stave off the inevitable end to life. America's medical decisions are rooted in this tradition.

Spending huge amounts of money on the process of dying has been part of our way of life for decades. A 1964 study showed that the median bill for hospital and other institutional expenses of sick adults who died were almost three times those of sick adults who did not die.[14, 15]

A 1970 study conducted at Massachusetts General Hospital concluded intensive care costs seem to be inversely related to the probability of patient survival. In other words, the more money we spend the more likely the patient is to die.[16]

A study of billed charges of the last two weeks of life of patients terminally ill with malignant disease showed the cost was 10.5 times greater in a hospital than at home. Diagnostic and therapeutic services were given to nearly all patients until the day of death.[17]

A 1984 study of Medicare beneficiaries in Colorado who died in 1978 found that average Medicare reimbursements for enrollees who died were six times the average reimbursements for enrollees who survived ($6,000 compared to $1,000).[15, 18]

A 1984 Blue Cross and Blue Shield Association study of cancer care for the terminally ill determined that expenditures averaged $21,219 for the terminal year and grew exponentially as death approached, with $6,161 being spent in the final month alone. The study included a shocking estimate: 205,000 people, representing about half of those who died of cancer, accounted for nearly 2 percent of the nation's entire health care bill.[19]

A health care root system once thought to be buried deep in the good earth of infinite resources has been exposed by a relentless erosion force, medical claims paid with thousands of IOU treasury instruments. An exposed root system will topple the tallest tree.

IV. Systemic Cynicism

Cynicism is self-defeating. It impairs the patient/physician teamwork needed to maintain or restore health. People who are perceived to make their living from another's misfortune are held in contempt. People who live life sheltered from the consequences of their own actions are resented.

Too many patients hold their doctors in contempt. Too many doctors resent their patients. This adversarial relationship has its problems. First among them is that physician/patient interactions are filled with doubt. Doubt breeds cynicism.

Our nation's model for health care builds cynicism into the system. The conceptual boundaries for our health care system are organized around the belief in powerful physicians and helpless patients.

The walnut shell provides an instructive metaphor. As the walnut develops, moisture and nutrients are trapped inside the new shell. The hardened shell protects the potential for a new tree as the seed matures. The sheltered seed can live a safe life for a long time but not forever. If the shell is not cracked the seed will rot. Eventually it will become hollow. The walnut shell is a boundary which must be broken for growth.

Our medical beliefs have a hard shell and they are a tough nut to crack. The shell promotes an internal technology and efficiency for which traditional medicine is justifiably famous. It is a conceptual boundary which simultaneously excludes data that would strengthen every prescribed treatment plan and reduce the price of every treatment outcome.

New beliefs threaten old beliefs. Old thought leaders will fight to the death to protect their ideals. New thought leaders who assault their position with overwhelming evidence will find neither cowardice nor retreat. Few industries welcome knowledge, however profound, which threatens their philosophical foundation. No matter. It is easy to illustrate our current belief system's flawed logic.

The process boundaries we set for the art of medicine closely resemble the ones we use for manufacturing (Figure 2.2). Symptoms are the specifications required to start treatment production. For a symptom to be a symptom it must be measurable. Specifically, it must be measured by a physical science. Chemistry, pathology, radiology, imaging, or histology are the gold standards used to determine the root cause of any given medical problem.

Once a symptom is quantified and a root cause is identified, production begins. Medical protocols are followed with precision. Technology, medical and surgical, is the primary tool of precision.

Medical process outputs are inspected. These outputs are misleadingly called outcomes. In 1990, the inspection of medical outputs often amounts to a superficial review of perpetual treatment (Figure 2.3). The twentieth

```
         MANUFACTURING PROCESS
    \      \      |      /      /
     \      \     |     /      /
      \      SPECIFICATION(S) /
       \      \    |    /    /
        ↘      ↘   ↓   ↙    ↙
        ┌─────────────────────┐
        │                     │
        │     PRODUCTION      │
        │                     │
        └─────────────────────┘
        ↙      ↙   ↓   ↘    ↘
       /      /    |    \    \
      /      INSPECTION(S)   \
     /      /     |     \     \
    ↙      ↙      ↓      ↘     ↘
```

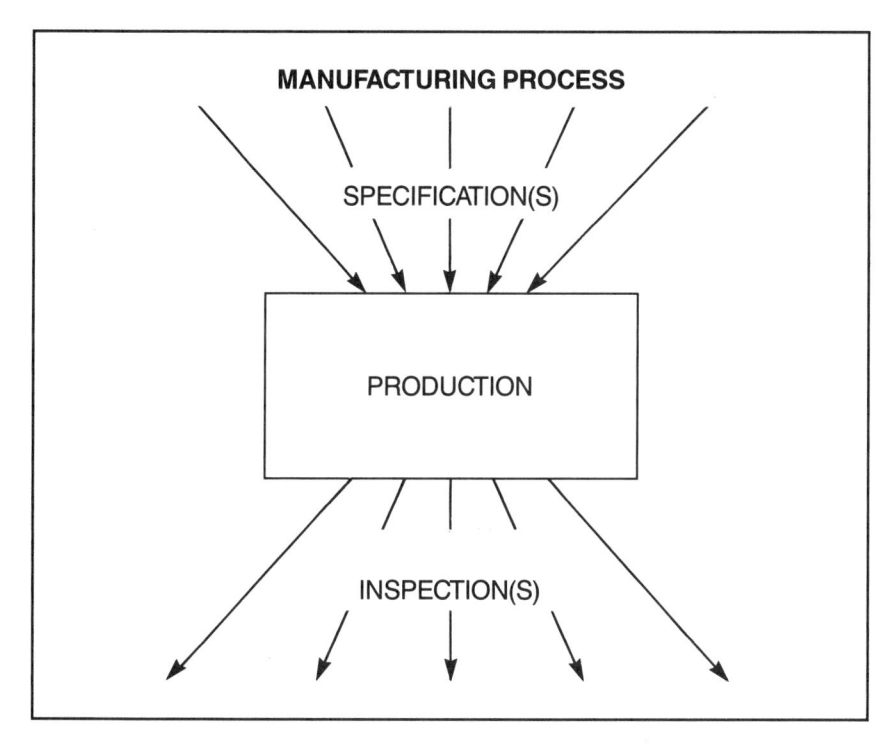

Figure 2.2 Process boundaries for the art of medicine resemble those set for manufacturing. *Adapted with permission of McGraw-Hill from Juran's Quality Control Handbook,* Fourth Edition, *page 6.20.*

century medical arts process is not designed to prevent problems from recurring. Medical science, as we know it, is designed to patch and mend. In one sense, medical marketing is designed to repeatedly cycle the customer through the health care system. For a few, more cycles just means more profit.

Enlightened manufacturers know every process, including the medical art's process, is actually an extended process. An extended process involves two additional vital elements, raw materials and outcome.

A painter cannot be expected to produce a masterpiece with mildewed canvas and dried paints. A physician cannot be expected to produce a satisfactory outcome when he or she treats a patient whose body cannot be healed through mechanical medical intervention. Yet we do expect the physician to produce good outcomes, with satisfied and healthy patients.

This is an unreasonable expectation. Any artist given defective or poor quality materials will produce work which delivers less than a satisfactory

MANUFACTURING PROCESS

SUPPLIER(S) OF RAW MATERIALS

INPUT(S)

PROCESS(ES)

PRODUCT(S)

CUSTOMER REACTION(S)

MEDICAL ARTS PROCESS 1990

HEALTH STATUS

SYMPTOMS OF DISEASE

MEDICAL DIAGNOSIS AND INTERVENTION

SHORT TERM RECOVERY

PERPETUAL TREATMENT

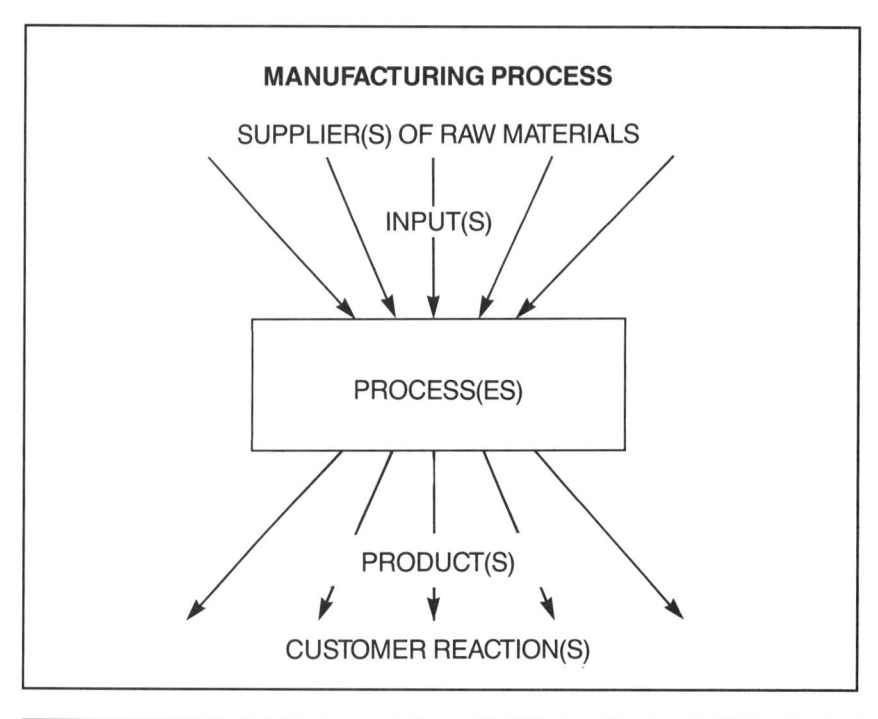

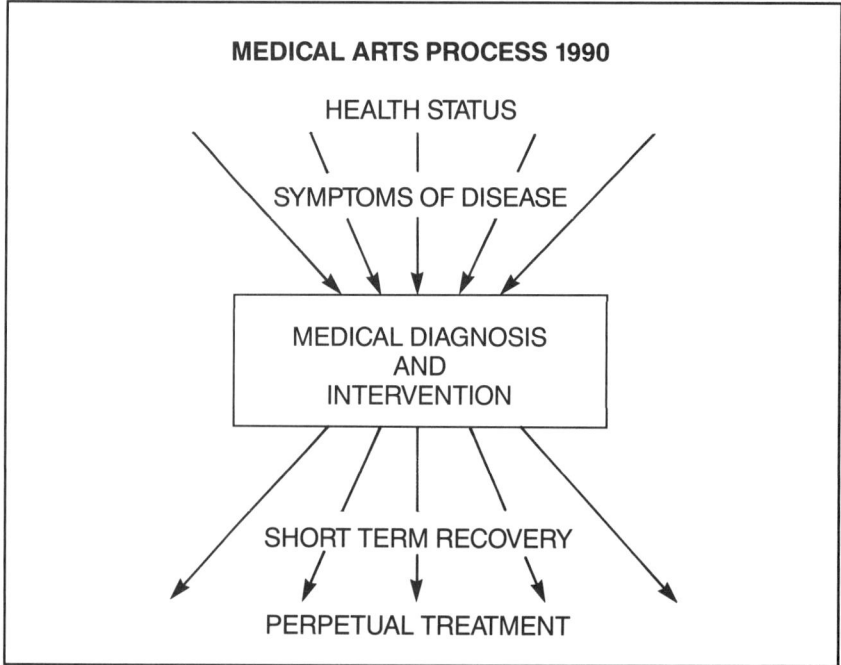

Figure 2.3 The inspection of outcomes can be a superficial review of perpetual treatment. *Adapted with permission of McGraw-Hill from* Juran's Quality Control Handbook, Fourth Edition, *page 6.20.*

outcome. It a painter has each image slashed before the paint dries, the painter will soon cease to paint well.

So it is for physicians who are asked to heal patients who continue to smoke, who abuse alcohol and other drugs, who eat a high fat diet, who refuse to exercise and who reject psychotherapy, biofeedback, relaxation, and meditation as treatment options. The task is impossible.

REFERENCES

1. Amler, R.W., and H.B. Dull, *Closing the Gap: The Burden of Unnecessary Illness.* New York: Oxford Press, 1987.

2. Juran, J.M. *Managerial Breakthrough.* New York: McGraw-Hill, 1964.

3. National Institute of Health. "Lowering Blood Cholesterol to Prevent Heart Disease." Bethesda, MD: GPO, 1985.

4. Surgeon General. *Healthy People: The Surgeon General's Report on Health Promotion and Disease Prevention.* Washington, DC: GPO, 1979.

5. Wechsler, H., E.H. Kasey, D. Thum, and H.W. Demone. "Alcohol Level and Home Accidents." *Public Health Reports* (1984): 1043-1969.

6. Department of Transportation. "Report of NHTSA Task Force to Analyze the Effectiveness of Various Restraint Systems." Washington DC: GPO, 1984.

7. Miller, N.S., M.S. Gold, and R.L. Millman. "Cocaine." *American Family Physician* 39, No. 2: (1989) 115-20.

8. Moore, R.D., L. Bone, and G. Geller. "Prevalence, Detection and Treatment of Alcoholism in Hospitalized Patients." *JAMA* 261, No. 3 (1989): 403-407.

9. American Agenda, Inc. Report, 1989, p. 272, Book of the Month Club.

10. Regier, D.A. and R.M.A. Hirschfeld. "The NIMH Depression Awareness, Recognition, and Treatment Program: Structure, Aims, and Scientific Basis."

11. Christopherson, B., and C. Pfeiffer. "Varying the Timing of Information to Alter Preoperative Anxiety and Postoperative Recovery in Cardiac Surgery Patients." *Heart and Lung* 9, No. 5 (1980): 854-861.

12. Stoudemire, A. "Depression in the Medically Ill." In *Psychiatry,* Vol. 2, edited by J.O. Cavenar. New York: Lippincott, 1985.

13. Quill, T.E. "Somatization Disorder, One of Medicine's Blind Spots," *JAMA* 254, No. 21 (1985): 3075-3079.

14. Timmer, E.J., and M.G. Kovar. "Expenses for Hospital and Institutional Care During the Last Year of Life for Adults Who Died in 1964 and 1965." *Vital and Health Statistics,* Series 22, No. 11 (March 1971).

15. Scitovsky, A.A. "The High Cost of Dying: What Do the Data Show?" *Health and Society* 62, No. 4 (1984): 591-608.

16. Civetta, J.M. "The Inverse Relationship Between Cost and Survival." *Journal of Surgical Research* 14 (1973): 265-269.

17. Bloom, B.S., and P.D. Kissick. "Home and Hospital Costs of Terminal Illness." *Medical Care* 18, No. 5 (1980): 560-564.

18. McCall, N. "Utilization and Costs of Medicare Services by Beneficiaries in the Last Year of Life." *Medical Care* 22, No. 4 (1984): 329-342.

19. Long, S. H., J. O. Gibbs, and J. P. Crozier. "Medical Expenditures of Terminal Cancer Patients During the Last Year of Life." *Inquiry* 21 (Winter 1984): 315-327.

3
THE QUALITY APPROACH

Each obstacle raises challenging questions. Each question amplifies the chaos which pervades our health care system.

Is it realistic to think that we can afford quality care for everyone? Is it possible to stop people from making themselves sick? Do people get sick because the system is a failure? Are health care givers guilty or guiltless?

No wonder our nation and the world puzzle over the problem of delivering quality health care. It is our good fortune that the mathematics and philosophy which have become known as World Class Manufacturing provide clear direction.

The confusing set of problems health care providers face today are no less perplexing than the task Walter A. Shewhart and his team faced at the Bell Telephone Laboratories in the 1920s and 1930s. They were expected to provide the leadership needed to initiate the mass production and distribution of telephones. The quality of their thinking and the quality of their work determined the quality of our nation's first electronic communication system.

An infinite number of variables seemed beyond human control. Scores of questions, most of which had never been asked before, needed to be answered quickly and correctly.

Was it realistic to link every person in the country together by telephone? Could the nation afford the idea? Could quality characteristics be operationally defined? Could a common set of quality values be agreed upon? Could unskilled labor produce the most technologically complex instrument ever invented? Could the product be produced profitably?

Could factory workers, doctoral-level statisticians, and engineers learn to cooperate and collaborate? How much product variation would be acceptable? How much variation would result from common causes? How much variation would come from special causes?

Despite the obstacles and the questions posed, an affordable, dependable, reliable telephone was mass produced. It provided a standardized communication link for the entire population of a developing nation. It was a monumental job. It was accomplished profitably.

The telephone system is a tribute to the continuous quality improvement theories of Shewhart. A statistician by profession, Shewhart was also a first-rate philosopher.

Shewhart's original thinking and practical approach defined a quintessential approach to quality and the quality improvement process. First he defined the three primary steps to statistical process control: specification, production, and judgment of quality (Figure 3.1).

STEP I	STEP II	STEP III
Specification ⟶	Production ⟶	Judgment of Quality

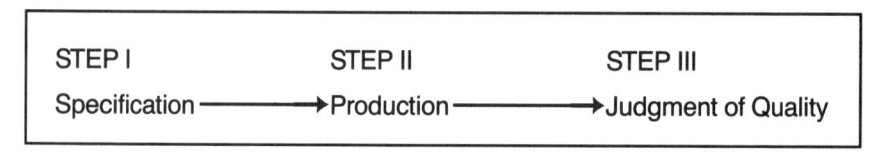

Figure 3.1 Three primary steps to statistical process control. *Used with permission of the American Society of Quality Control. Walter Shewhart,* Statistical Method from the Viewpoint of Quality Control, *page 45.*

Shewhart's astute observation of the importance of original data sequence in this process was profound. In *Statistical Method from the Viewpoint of Quality Control*[1] he wrote:

> I think it is particularly important to note that the third step cannot be taken by simply inspecting the quality of the objects* as objects, but instead must be taken by inspecting the objects in a sequence ordered in relation to the production** process. In fact, these three steps must go in a circle instead of in a straight line, as shown schematically in Figure 3.2. It may be helpful to think of the three steps in the mass production process as steps in the scientific method.

---

*Substitute the word disease for the word object to see the relevance of this quote.
**Substitute the word health for production in this sentence.

In this sense, specification, production, and inspection correspond respectively to making a hypothesis, carrying out an experiment, and testing the hypothesis. The three steps constitute a dynamic scientific process of acquiring *knowledge* [emphasis added]. From this viewpoint, it might be better to show them as forming a sort of spiral gradually approaching a circular path which would represent the idealized case where no evidence is found in Step III to indicate a need for changing the specification (or scientific hypothesis) no matter how many times we repeat the three steps. Mass production viewed in this way constitutes a continuing and self-corrective method for making the most efficient use of raw and fabricated materials.

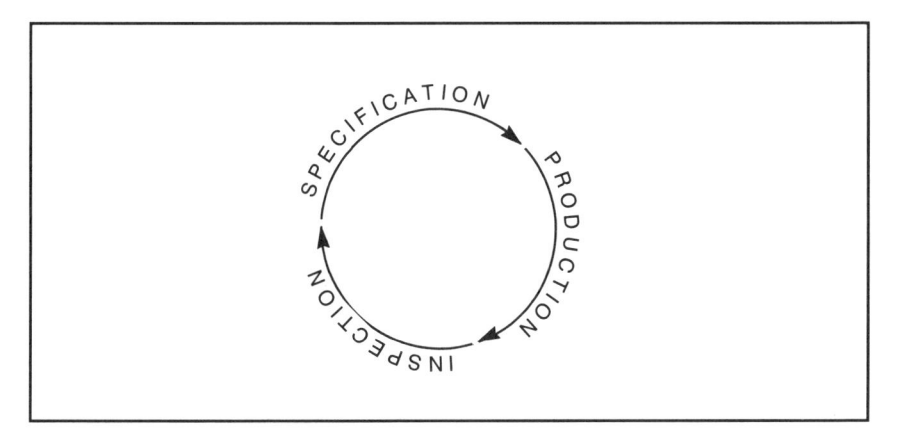

Figure 3.2 The three primary steps of statistical process control move in a circle. *Used with permission of the American Society for Quality Control. Walter Shewhart,* Statistical Method from the Viewpoint of Quality Control, *page 45.*

In the *Economic Control of Quality of Manufactured Product*[2] he summarized, "The practical problem involves induction instead of deduction."

Induction is a method of reasoning or mathematical proof in which a conclusion is reached about all members of a given set by examining just a few members of the set. Deduction, the opposite of induction, is the process of reasoning from a known principle to an unknown, from the general to the specific or from a premise to a conclusion.

Shewhart's three-part cycle evolved into a four-part process. He labeled the quadrants of this scientific process Plan, Do, Study, Act.[3] When W. Edwards Deming* introduced the Shewhart Cycle to Japan in 1950 it became Plan, Do, Check, Act (Figure 3.3). Deming gave credit where credit was due but the cycle's name was changed to the Deming Cycle.[4] This cycle is a keystone in World Class Manufacturing's foundation.

---

*Deming was a colleague and remains a student of Shewhart. He has firmly established himself as a world-renowned champion of quality. He has received many awards, including the Shewhart Medal from the American Society for Quality Control.

We can only speculate on the relationship between Shewhart's theory of process and that of his contemporary, Albert Einstein. Einstein wrote in his book *Relativity*[5]:

> From a systematic theoretical point of view, we may imagine the process of evolution of an empirical science to be a continuous process of induction... it is as it were, a purely empirical enterprise.

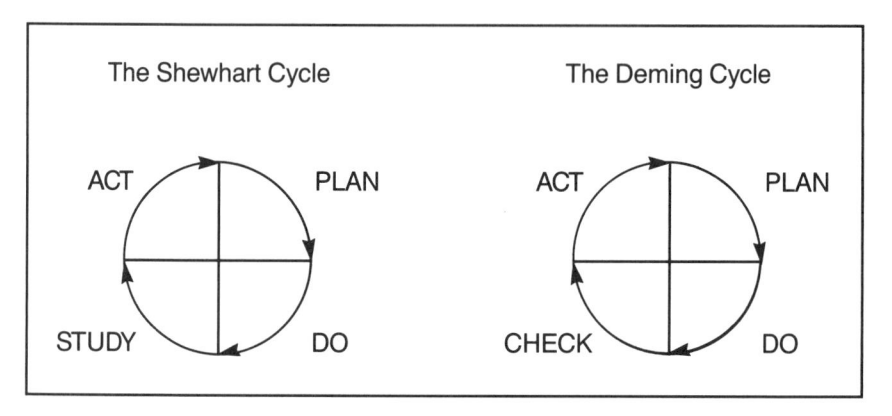

Figure 3.3 Shewhart cycle vs Deming cycle.

Surely it is more than coincidence that Shewhart's theory, taken in its entirety, represents the classically balanced interplay between induction, empiricism, intuition, and deductive thought that Einstein referred to when he described the development of an exact science.

Shewhart used the word knowledge in an epistemological sense. Epistemology is the theory or science which investigates the origin, nature, methods, and limits of knowledge. It is a rewarding philosophical specialty. Epistemology requires patience plus an ability and will to understand abstract ideas.

Shewhart's theory of statistical process control was greatly influenced by a system of philosophic thought called conceptual pragmatism. C. I. Lewis, a philosophy professor from Harvard, published a book about this system in 1929 entitled, *Mind and the World Order, Outline of a Theory of Knowledge*[6] It is referenced a number of times in Shewhart's work.* Shewhart's logical extension of Lewis' thinking is unmistakable.

Lewis took the traditional grounds of a priori (logically first) truth to task in the preface of his book when he boldly overstated, "Traditional grounds of a priori truth have been perforce, abandoned."[6]

---

*Shewhart frequently cites C. I. Lewis' book *Mind and The World Order* in his second book. On pages 254 and 393, Lewis cited Einstein's book *Relativity*. We think the relationship between Einstein's ideas and Shewhart's thinking is striking.

An elementary understanding of the epistemological concept, a priori, is the first building block in a quality approach to health care because the core of the quality idea revolves around the continuous discovery, management, and practical application of new knowledge. A combination of several dictionary definitions for a priori clarifies the meaning of this term.

In philosophy a priori means prior to. A priori concepts furnish the basis of experience. A priori is based on theory instead of experience or experiment. It is presumptive, without or before examination. A priori is deductive, relating to or derived by reasoning from self-evident propositions.

According to Professor Lewis[6]:

> The a priori is not a material truth, delimiting or delineating the content of experience as such, but is definitive or analytic in its nature...
>
> Since it is a truth about our own interpretive attitude, it imposes no limitation upon future possibilities of experience; that is a priori which we can maintain in the face of all experience, come what will.

A priori provides a conceptual framework. It summarizes and categorizes past experience. For example, at one time it was a scientific a priori assumption that our earth was the center of our planetary system. This a priori was once a handy way of looking at our world as we knew it.

Lewis elaborates on the value of a priori thinking (deductive, presumptive reasoning):

> ...deduction in general, which although perhaps inevitable to an earlier day, is quite unwarranted. According to this view the logically first principles, or presuppositions, are self-evident axioms which, through the process of deduction, shed the glory of their certainty on all propositions deduced from them...
>
> The supposed necessity or logical indispensability, of presuppositions most frequently turns out to be nothing more significant than lack of imagination and ingenuity.

This is courageous, lucid thinking. It is the pivotal epistemological point of view which distinguishes Shewhart's brilliant approach to quality. The collective wisdom of Einstein,[5] Lewis,[6] and Shewhart[1,2] provides a specific answer for those of us who ponder the question, "How can I build quality into the health care process?" The writings of a genius, a philosopher, and a statistician answers, "Think clearly and reason statistically."

To think clearly means to think independently and freely, unimpaired by the bias and taboos of presuppositions. All knowledge is relative. Einstein explained why knowledge must have a well-defined frame of reference. Lewis explained how knowledge, even when it is firing on all 12 cylinders, is probable only. Shewhart's statistical methods turned probability calculus into an easy-to-use tool.

A priori assumptions are seductive. If we don't keep our wits about us they cloud our thinking with illusion. They make us carefree about what we "know." A priori can fool us into taking knowledge for granted when we must never take knowledge for granted. Scientific thought and quality thinking require inquisitive minds which relentlessly raise the question, Why? Why? Why? Why? Why?

The folk story about the emperor's new clothes is a timeless example of deductions logically made from a flawed a priori assumption. The thinking and behavior of the royal subjects were illuminated by a wide-eyed child not yet indoctrinated by a common presumption: The emperor was clothed. Conceptual pragmatism and statistical reasoning bring today's medical model into the same light of day.

The traditional medical model's a priori assumption is that there is an organic genesis for all disease. We have allowed this assumption to control our beliefs about how we get sick and how we get well. We take it for granted that if someone is sick there must first be something wrong with his or her body.

Medicine's self-evident, logically first conclusion has provided a superb conceptual framework for the health sciences up to this point in time. Einstein pays a compliment to any theory which has served humanity so well[5]:

> No fairer destiny could be allotted to any physical theory than that it should point out the way to the introduction of a more comprehensive theory, in which it lives on as a limiting case.[5]

Medicine's first logically deduced conclusion about an illness is that the body's chemistry or physiology must be repaired. Therefore, medical intervention to adjust the body's chemistry or surgical intervention to change the physiology is the indispensable prescription of choice. This thinking turns out to be much too narrow.

A substantial body of empirical evidence suggests the genesis of the *disease process* has much to do with thoughts, emotions, and lifestyle. The preferred prescription must be a combined approach of lifestyle education (with a pronounced emphasis on tobacco use, and drug and alcohol misuse), psychotherapy, medical treatment, and, when necessary, surgical treatment.

Health care providers need to be skilled in a multidisciplinary approach to treatment. They also need to know when and where to apply it. Taking action on any process without an awareness of its state of statistical control is tantamount to tampering. Tampering does more harm than good. Tampering is contrary to the first charge of every medical practitioner, "Do no harm."

Shewhart's theory of statistical process control empowers care givers with a powerful conceptual tool, the control chart. This tool can help care givers determine the when and the where of health care intervention. Shewhart[1] says the idea of control involves "action taken to achieve a desired end."

The control chart is a masterpiece. It is built on the solid ground of arithmetic, formal distribution theory, empirical observation, and inductive reasoning. It establishes the ways and means of making better use of past experience.

Arithmetic (formal distribution theory and its summary of probabilities and variation) is, according to C. I. Lewis[6]:

> an a priori truth of concepts which have concrete denotation...Arithmetic depends *in toto* upon the operation of counting or correlating a procedure which can be carried out in any world containing identifiable things.
>
> It is because this is true that arithmetic is a priori. Its laws prevent *nothing*; they are compatible with anything which happens or conceivably could happen in nature.

Professor Lewis[6] repeatedly emphasized the importance of mathematics to knowledge and he stated flatly, "There is no knowledge without interpretation."

This notion rang true for the statistician Shewhart[1] who extended Lewis' thinking when he wrote, "Every interpretation involves a prediction."

Shewhart's picture is worth a thousand words concerning the relationship between the a priori of arithmetic and the sequential order of empirical data. The control chart is built on a truly reliable, neutral a priori conceptual frame of reference. It frames discreet data points in the order in which they occur. This order is necessary to inductive reasoning. The control chart makes accurate predictions within the limits of probability possible (Figure 3.4).

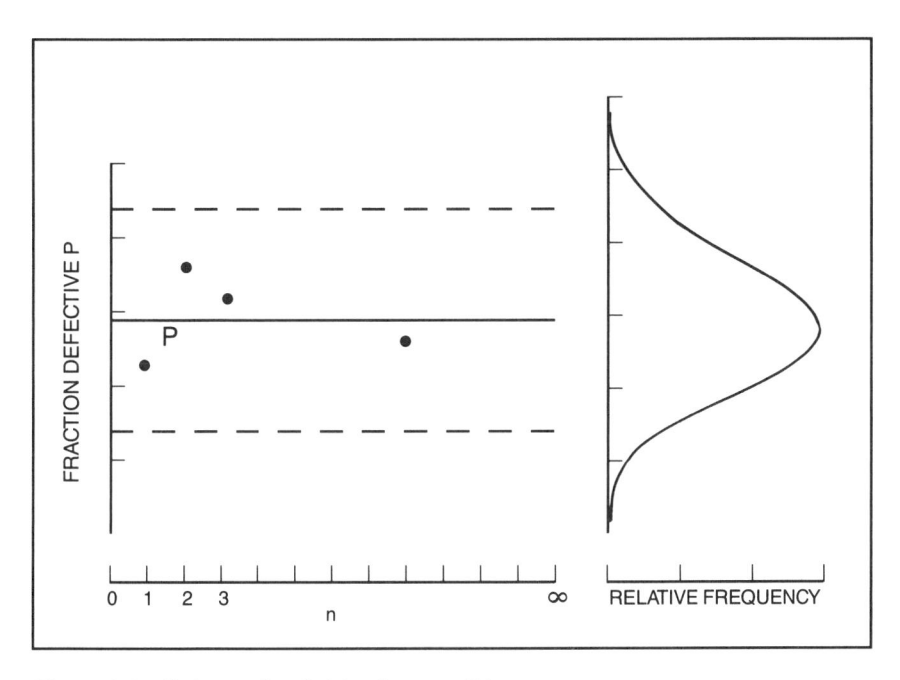

Figure 3.4 Schematic of objective condition.

Although Shewhart's guiding philosophy was complex, grade school math is sufficient to understand the fundamental statistical theory required to construct and interpret a control chart. A simplified statistical experiment using your time, a pair of dice, graph paper, and a straightedge gives a good first lesson.

1. Roll two dice 5,000 times. Record each number rolled on a check sheet as illustrated.

```
 2 XXXXXXXXXX
 3 XXXXXXXXXXXXXXX
 4 XXXXXXXXXXXXXXXXXXXX
 5 XXXXXXXXXXXXXXXXXXXXXXXXX
 6 XXXXXXXXXXXXXXXXXXXXXXXXXXXXXX
 7 XXXXXXXXXXXXXXXXXXXXXXXXXXXXXXXXXXX
 8 XXXXXXXXXXXXXXXXXXXXXXXXXXXXXX
 9 XXXXXXXXXXXXXXXXXXXXXXXXX
10 XXXXXXXXXXXXXXXXXXXX
11 XXXXXXXXXXXXXXX
12 XXXXXXXXXX
```

2. Using graph paper, X out one square for each 10 times a given number appears to create a histogram. Your histogram will resemble the bell-shaped curve in Shewhart's illustration. The highest cell, the most frequently occurring number in the histogram, is seven. This number is called the mode. In our experiment this number is also the mean or average and the median.

The average of a group of numbers is calculated by adding the sum of all numbers rolled and dividing by the total number of rolls.

$$\frac{35,000}{5,000} = 7$$

The median is the dividing line where 50 percent of all data points fall above and 50 percent fall below (Figure 3.5).

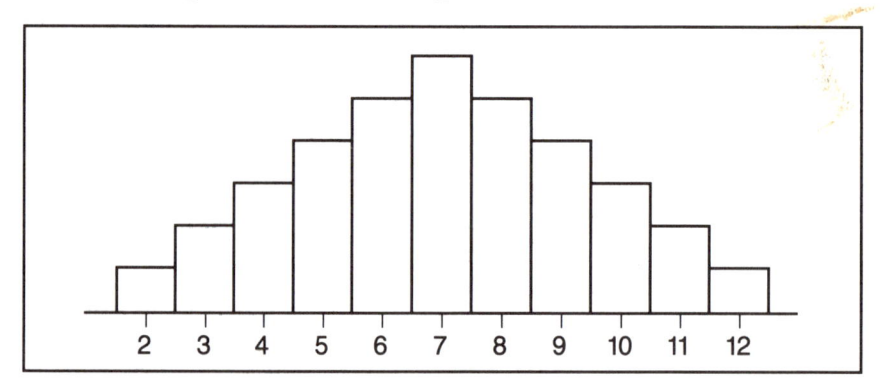

Figure 3.5 Histogram constructed from dice rolls.

A normal bell-shaped curve often is divided into six equal sections. Figure 3.6 summarizes the percentage of points which fall in each section and the probability of data points falling within those boundaries in successive trials.

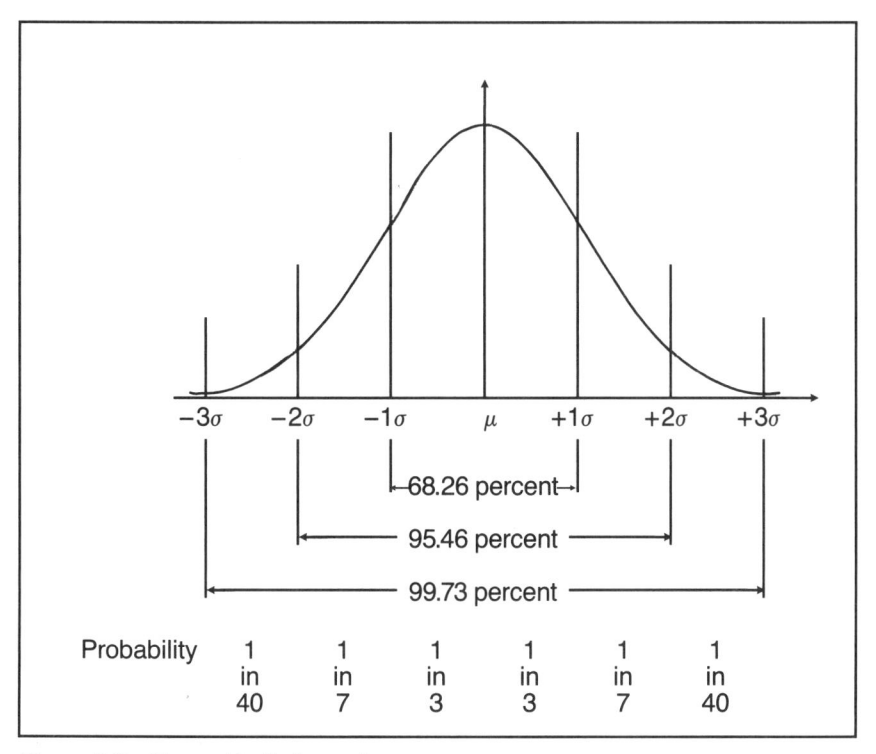

Figure 3.6 Normal bell-shaped curve.

3. Using another piece of graph paper label 12 lines, 2 to 12 as illustrated. Mark the upper control limit, 12, with a dotted line. Mark the lower control limit, 2, with a dotted line. Using a straightedge, draw a solid center line across the mean, 7 (Figure 3.7).

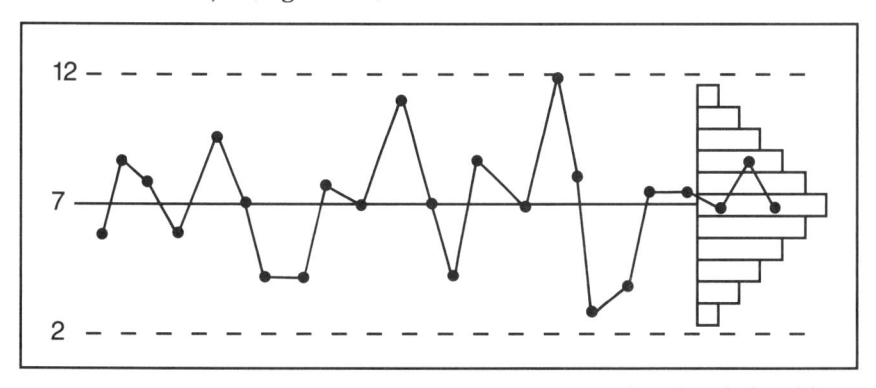

Figure 3.7 Random dice rolls plotted in sequence over time, in relationship to a histogram of the dice roll population.

4. Roll the dice 25 times. Record each number by marking a dot on the grid mark as shown. Connect dot one to dot two and so on until the entire pattern of variation is visible.

Congratulations. You have just determined the state of statistical control for a simple, finite process—the roll of the dice. It is a stable process with only random variation. The process output can be accurately predicted within a range of normal probabilities, 2 to 12.

If any number 0, 1, or 13 and above occurred you would immediately know a "special cause" had changed the process. Perhaps only one die was thrown or maybe three dice were being used (Figure 3.8A).

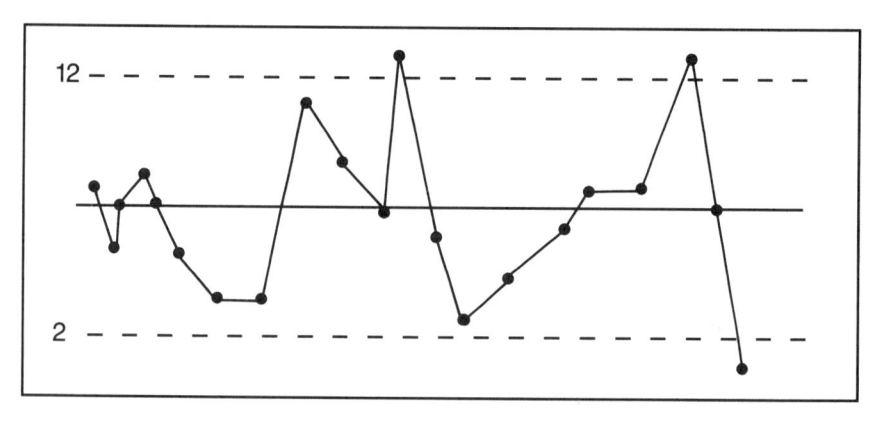

Figure 3.8A Evidence of out of control for dice roll. Are two dice being rolled? Is one die being rolled? Is the reported roll accurate?

If a nonrandom pattern appeared, for instance, four out of five rolls producing 2 or 12, you would also suspect a "special cause." The dice may be loaded or the person collecting data might be fibbing (Figure 3.8B).

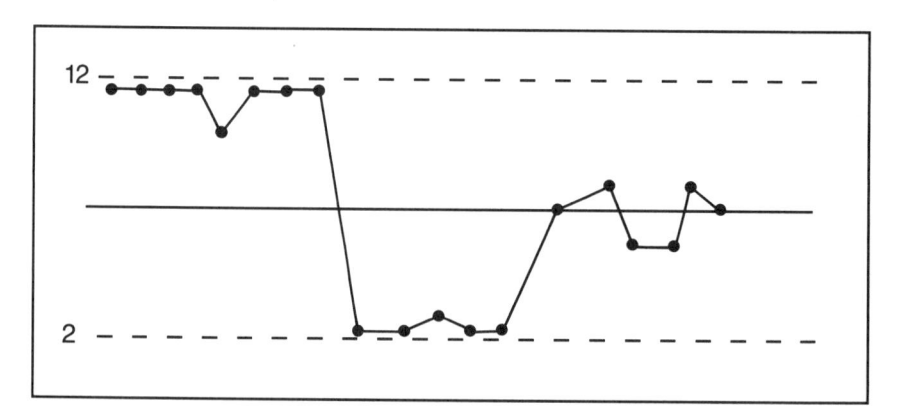

Figure 3.8B Evidence of out of control dice rolls. Are the dice loaded? Are the data reports accurate?

If you wanted to get a 0, a 1, or a 13, 14, etc., you could "control" the process by including those variables in the process. If you wanted to return the process to its original state of statistical control you would have to remove those causes. If you wanted to reduce the variation in the original process you may want to use one die.

In order to take the proper control action to get the desired result, one must first determine a given process' state of statistical control. If we fail to determine the state of statistical control for a process, we have no way of determining whether an event is a result of random chance or part of a pattern. If we take action without this knowledge, we risk overcontrolling or undercontrolling the process. Overcontrol and undercontrol are tampering, and tampering creates chaos. Chaos is a statistical word used to describe an unpredictable, out-of-control process. A bundle of chaotic processes creates a chaotic system.

Shewhart thought of statistical control as a never-to-be achieved ideal state. He determined that the best approach to this ideal was to minimize errors of overcontrol and undercontrol. Control chart formulas are tools which can help us determine a process' state of statistical control without knowing the limits and capabilities of the process in advance. In effect, Shewhart invented predictive statistics. By recording the order of occurrence of data on the chart, we can determine whether a process is in control, i.e., random chance is responsible for all variation, or out of control, i.e., special or assignable causes are influencing the process.

Data order sequence is of the utmost importance to predictive statistics. Deming[1] drew attention to this point in a 1988 foreword to Shewhart's statistical methods book:

> A record of observations must accordingly contain all the information that anyone might need in order to make his own prediction.
>
> This information will include not merely numerical data, but also (for example): the names of observers, the type of apparatus or measurement system used, a description of materials used, the temperature and humidity, a description of efforts taken to reduce error, the side effects and other external factors that in the judgment of the expert in the subject matter may be helpful for use of the results.
>
> Omission from data (as of a test or a run of production) of information on the order of the observations may well bury for purposes of prediction (i.e., for planning) nearly all the information that there is in the test. Any symmetric function loses the information that is contained in the order of observation. Thus, the mean, standard deviation—in fact any moment—is in most applications inefficient, as it causes the loss of all information as contained in the order of observation. A distribution is another example of a symmetric function. Original data plotted in order of production may provide much more information than is contained in the distribution.
>
> Dr. Shewhart was well aware that the statisticians' levels of significance furnish no measure of belief in a prediction. Probability has use; tests of significance do not.[1]

The natural law of large numbers expressed in a normal distribution curve provides the ideal frame for evaluating the randomness and non-randomness of variation. At three standard deviations above and below the mean 99.73 percent of all expected occurrences are included.

Two of the four important characteristics of original data Shewhart said needed to be considered in the presentation of data are represented in a control chart; numbers representing numeric values of measurements and the order in which the numbers were taken are summarized. The log which accompanies a control chart describes the conditions under which each measurement was made, including a description of the operation of measurement and a summary of the human element or observer. When original data include all four characteristics, we have the power to make accurate predictions.

For example, the chart in Figure 3.8C graphs 24 data points of an individual's potassium level. Potassium levels are of particular interest to patients who are taking a medication which robs potassium from their body. If a person's potassium level is not correct, muscles, including the heart muscle, cease to function properly (Figure 3.8C).

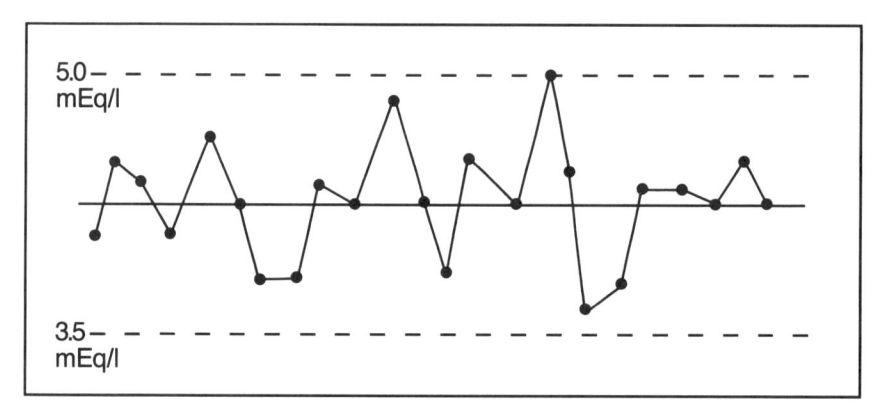

Figure 3.8C Normal variation of potassium levels.

All the points fall within the normal range of variation considered to be healthy. The distribution of the points indicates that the process is in statistical control. All data points in this process arise from a system of chance causes. No one data point has any more significance than any other.

The following control chart (Figure 3.8D) indicates the presence of several assignable, or special, causes which fall outside the range of what one would expect from a healthy system of chance causes. The special causes evidenced represent life-threatening events.

The practical problem of predicting and controlling the immediate future of this process first requires the elimination of special (assignable) causes. A long sequence usually is required to remove assignable causes or, when

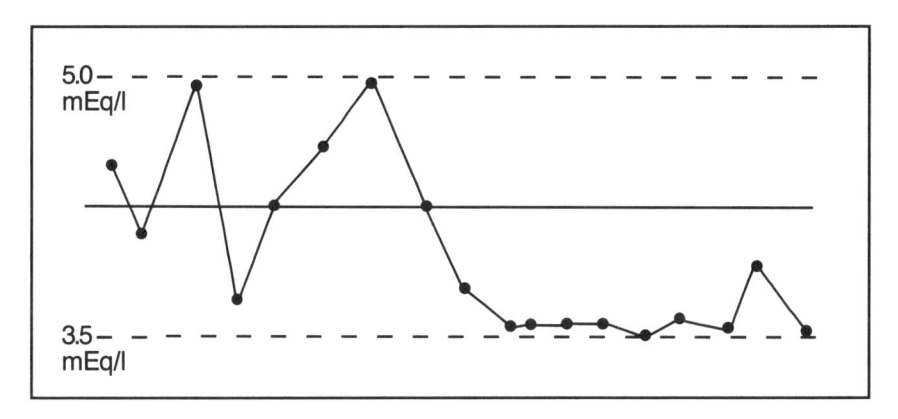

Figure 3.8D Nonrandom variation of potassium levels.

desired, to incorporate them into a process. Once a process is in statistical control, maximum control can be achieved and variation can be continuously reduced. We can take action to achieve our desired result.

The reasoning of statistical process control is inductive. Mathematical proof is an output of a control chart. This proof confirms or disproves the hypothesis of the experiment. It tells us whether our belief about reality was true or false. Inductive reasoning must be done relative to the boundaries of a specified observed process. Each and every process is distinctive unto itself. All knowledge is relative.

Obviously, action taken to remove a special cause must be substantially different from action taken to change an entire system of common causes. Shewhart's control chart is the best tool available for deciding which control action is needed. Knowledge of variation and the proper use of control charts discourages tampering. Tampering is treating a common cause of variation as if it were a special cause or treating a special cause of variation as if it were a common cause.

The quality approach to health care must include statistical methods from the viewpoint of quality control. This will minimize chaos and the losses which arise from tampering. The quality approach must also include appropriate medical science, cognitive therapy, and health education.

Genuine teamwork is a new idea in health care. Traditionally orders have been given by a power figure. Things are not so different from the way Hippocrates practiced his art 2,000 years ago.

Things change.

Teamwork, cooperation, and collaboration are essential to the quality approach. The medical doctor knows the most about medicine. The patient knows the most about his or her lifestyle. Psychologists know the most about behavior. Nurses know the most about nursing people back to health. This knowledge is potent when it is combined. It can be combined when each team member respects the expertise of the other.

Physicians, psychologists, nurse educators,* and patients are peers on every treatment team. Each must have equal influence on treatment decisions. This partnership sets boundaries so cynicism is placed outside the system and not built into it.

A quality approach, World Class Health Care, acknowledges the importance of raw materials and health status. Patients are expected to contribute healthy lifestyles or they must accept less than optimal outcomes at higher than necessary costs.

World Class Health Care endorses the wisdom of multidisciplinary diagnostic and treatment approaches. Statistics are the international language of quality. Every input of symptoms requires a comprehensive medical science, behavioral science, and lifestyle assessment. Diagnostic data can be expected to uncover all potential root causes of an illness including self-destructive thinking, dangerous health habits, depression, alcoholism, and drug addiction. Diagnostics can be expected to expose more than chemistry profiles. They must uncover and describe the profiles which predict illness and violence.

In a World Class Health Care system good outcomes, resilient good health, and patient satisfaction are necessarily the shared responsibility of all parties. Except in rare instances of malicious intent or gross misjudgment, the notion of malpractice based strictly on outcome disappears because malpractice assumes some one person is at fault.

Deming[4] estimates that more than 94 percent of outcome problems reside in the process and not the people who are part of the process. This claim is easily verified with a simple Shewhart experiment. Using the pen of your choice, please print the letter A in the following blanks. Do your best!

_____ _____ _____ _____ _____ _____ _____ _____

It should come as no surprise that you failed to replicate the A described in the experiment directions. You can also see each letter varies slightly from the others. Ink, paper, time of day, lighting, concentration, hand preference, or the efficient substitution of a pencil all cause variation. Variation is a fact of life. Everything is one of a kind.

A physician can no more be held personally accountable for an optimal outcome than the writer can be blamed for inconsistent work. Hundreds of process variables are beyond control beginning with the patient's health status. An entire system of chance causes and related processes can and must be brought under control before reliable quality outcomes can be asked for or expected.

Regrettably, the late twentieth century medical arts focus on crisis management instead of process improvement. Consequently, medical centers play to a full house.

---

*In the context of quality care, nurse educator means any registered nurse or clinical nurse practitioner. Patient education and teaching must join nursing care as primary nursing responsibilities.

REFERENCES

1. Shewhart, W.A. *Statistical Method from the Viewpoint of Quality Control.* Mineola, NY: Dover Publications, Inc., 1986.

2. Shewhart, W.A. *Economic Control of Quality of Manufactured Product.* New York: Macmillan, Van Nostrand, 1931. Commemorative reissue Milwaukee: ASQC Quality Press, 1980.

3. Scholtes, P. *The Team Handbook.* Madison, WI: Joiner and Associates, 1988.

4. Deming, W.E. *Out of the Crisis.* Cambridge: Massachusetts Institute of Technology, 1988.

5. Einstein, A. *Relativity.* New York: Crown Publishers, 1916.

6. Lewis, C.I. *Mind and the World Order: Outline of a Theory of Knowledge.* New York: Dover Press, 1956.

4
CAST OF CHARACTERS

The cast of our nation's health care melodrama reaches from the President of the United States to the newest born baby in America. Three central roles are played out in hospitals every day of the year: the patient, the physician, and the administrator. Each has good intentions. Each can fall victim to the forces of an out-of-control system.

Everyone has been or knows someone who has been a hospital patient. We are familiar with their points of view, fears, frustration, and anger.

Illness eventually introduces each of us to a physician. Every patient has met a doctor; few are fortunate enough to count one as a personal friend.

Hospital administrators are unfamiliar and invisible. There are fewer than 6,000 hospital-based chief executive officers in a nation of 250 million people. They must allocate scarce, strategic resources. Their decisions must please the patients, physicians, and hospitals which pay their salaries.

Patient

You have been a patient many times. You learned that germs made people sick before you were old enough to walk. Germs were invisible. They struck without warning. You lived through the chicken pox, ear aches, strep throat, viral infections, and all the other childhood diseases. You learned that shots and pills made you well.

When you were sick you got to drink soda pop. You ate ice cream. You stayed home from school. You got extra attention.

Your early visits to the doctor's office are easy to remember. First you had to wait. You always waited because the doctor was a busy person. When the doctor got around to you he looked into your ears, eyes, and throat. He listened to your chest. He poked around your belly and thumped you on your back. He hit your knee with a rubber hammer. Sometimes he took a blood sample.

He didn't ask and you didn't tell him if you were happy or sad. He didn't ask and you didn't offer to do a pushup, a pull-up, or a sit-up. He didn't ask and you didn't say what you ate.

He gave you shots. He told you to take vitamin pills. He seemed to know more about you in 15 minutes than you knew about yourself.

You saw your first bacteria under a microscope in a ninth grade biology class. You learned how to grow paramecium in a petri dish.

You learned about the bubonic plague and smallpox in history class. You learned about cholera from a television show, *Wagon Train*. You learned about polio from the next door neighbor and his wheelchair. You figured out that hospitals were an absolute necessity.

When you went to the doctor's office for your junior school-year physical, you waited. Wasting time irritated you. You were missing practice. The weather was beautiful. You wondered why the doctor never kept his appointments on time.

The doctor's routine had changed a bit. His nurse now took the blood sample. She had you urinate in a bottle. She took your blood pressure.

He didn't ask and you didn't tell him if you were happy or sad. He didn't ask and you didn't say if you were drinking. You were relieved he didn't ask you any questions about sex. He didn't ask and you didn't say if you could walk a mile. He seemed too busy to listen. His sick patients must have needed him more than you did.

His self-confident manner no longer put you at ease. It intimidated you. You apologized for asking him about your itchy eyes and running nose. He said it was probably an allergy. He gave you pills to take care of the problem. They didn't work. He gave you allergy shots for two years and the problem was bearable.

When you went away to college, you stopped your shots. Your allergies seemed to disappear. When you went home at Thanksgiving, your allergies came back. You wondered if the family cat might be the problem.

In December you went in for a checkup. You waited for an hour before the nurse called you into the examining room. You waited in your underwear for another hour before the doctor came in to see you. He apologized for being late. "I had an emergency at the hospital."

He asked about your allergies. He laughed when you said you thought you were allergic to your family's cat. "Well you don't want to get rid of your cat, do you?"

He wasn't interested in small talk. He didn't ask you if you drank and he didn't ask if you smoked pot. It would have been none of his business anyway. He didn't ask you about your sex life and you didn't ask him about birth control. He didn't ask you what you ate. He didn't ask you about exercise. He didn't ask you if you were happy. He didn't ask you if you fibbed when you filled out the patient questionnaire. It didn't make any difference. You couldn't wait to get out of his office.

After you graduated from college you did what your parents did when they got sick. You treated your colds with drugstore remedies, chicken soup, and extra rest. You treated frustration with alcohol. Self-medication seemed to work pretty well.

Last Friday afternoon you went to your doctor's office for the first time in years. You had to. A friend had cut his hand on a broken glass. A six inch gash. You waited in his office for three hours. Finally, you left for a "Doc-in-the-Box store." For the first time in your life you didn't have to wait to see a doctor.

He sewed your friend up right away. $150. No questions asked. You made it home in time for *M*A*S*H* reruns.

Physician

You are a board-certified emergency physician. Put an MD after your name and be proud of it. It took you 24 years of education to get those initials and medicine is an honored profession.

The United States flies the only "Lear Jet" health care system on this planet. A distinguished, cut-throat competitive education earned you your pilot's wings. You make all in-flight decisions.

The killers of our past such as dysentery, diphtheria, and a host of other infectious diseases, are nonexistent. You and your colleagues can solve virtually any medical or surgical problem.

You have a right to expect a certain level of authority and a reasonably large paycheck. Your profession, your business, means the difference between a quality life, a disability, or an untimely death for your patients, your customers.

Medicine holds the same appeal it did when you were in grade school, although to be honest, the opportunity to acquire wealth prompted your career choice. For now, wealth taunts you from the distance. At age 33, your schooling has put you over $100,000 in debt. You are eight years of earned income behind your old college buddies.

The rules which govern your business are not well known to your patients. Your patients do not want to think of your practice as a business where goods and services are exchanged for a fee. Nevertheless, goods and services have always been exchanged in a doctor's office.

Since 1950, the fees physicians can charge for their antibiotics have grown in direct proportion to the availability of miraculous drugs. Lasers, computerized tomography, magnetic resonance imaging, and other physical science technologies have raised the market price of medical opinion and surgical skill. As an art, medicine commands private collector prices.

Every business has a pricing strategy. Your pricing strategy is aptly named the *Relative Value System (RVS)*. The RVS ranks each of your skills in order of their difficulty relative to the others. It establishes each skill's market value. The *RVS* is tied to a book entitled *International Classification of Diseases, 9th Revision, Clinical Modification (ICD-9-CM)*.[1] A separate volume of diagnostic criteria for psychological disorders, *Diagnostic and Statistical Manual 3rd Edition Revised (DSM-III-R)*,[2] is used only on rare occasions.

ICD-9-CM and *DSM-III-R* classify every medical model diagnosis known to man. *ICD-9-CM* serves as a biblical reference. It justifies a crucial medical science assumption; the etiology, the organic cause of a disease, is to be measured by the quantitative methodologies of physical science. Health care providers, insurance companies, and our government believe these measures are valid and reliable. They believe the *RVS, ICD-9-CM*, and when necessary, *DSM-III-R*, are the best tools to use in setting fair prices.

The *RVS* employs an elementary formula. One figure is chosen as a multiplier and one is chosen as a conversion factor. Conversion factors are progressive. They are proportional to the perceived expertise required to perform a given procedure. The *RVS* medical conversion figure averages $5 per unit. The standard *RVS* surgical conversion figure hovers near $60 per unit.

By multiplying a surgical conversion factor of $60 times a surgical multiplier of 20, the usual and customary surgical procedure charge equals $1,200. You can charge more if you think you do superior work and your patient or his or her insurance company is willing to pay for it.

A pre-med professor once drew a picture of the system's perverse incentives for you.

Potential per hour income for physicians

Office Work $100   Hospital Rounds $400   Surgical Work $3,000

The charge system presumes a higher degree of skill is required to intervene with surgery than is needed to intervene with medication. Patient education is easier and less dangerous than prescribing medication.

Therefore, it warrants the lowest level of remuneration.

History tells a different tale. Medicine and surgery are a relative breeze compared to the Herculean task of keeping people well. As a medical resident you spent time on patient education. Now it is not worth the effort. If you spend 30 minutes advising a patient not to drink a six-pack of beer when he is putting a new roof on his house you earn $25. If you wait until he wants you to set the leg he broke in a drunken fall, you earn $650.

Your patients and their insurers are blind to the built-in expense of *RVS* -based charges. Patients defer health maintenance. They won't pay a dime until something breaks down and neither will their insurance carriers.

The guy who postponed his diagnostic treadmill for fear of finding out his pain wasn't indigestion after all, is now recovering from the emergency surgery which followed his heart attack He saved $150. He spent $12,000.

The young woman who was afraid she would find a lump in her breast never did a breast self-examination. She shied away from a mammogram because her HMO insurance policy wouldn't pay the $65 charge. Now she's fighting for her 35-year-old life. She is also looking for a way to cover her $8,000 chemotherapy bill.

The system is less than perfect but it keeps the money in medicine. It can also take all the money out of it. It assumes, given medication and surgery, doctors can heal all comers regardless of their health histories and lifestyles. This seductive assumption keeps you exposed to a gigantic risk for an inevitable lawsuit. A single bad outcome can mean financial ruin. In our society, the larger the risk an individual is willing to assume, the greater the amount of money he or she has the right to dream about banking. Risk justifies your income.

The Judeo-Christian ethic runs deep in your blood. A God-fearing, God-loving people should do all things, at all times, under all circumstances to preserve every single human life. You are convinced health care is a right and not a privilege. People should have equal access to medical treatment. You like to work in the world's luxury hospitals. You take pride in the millions of dollars in medical technology and expertise which are a 911 phone call away for anyone who dials.

You love your job. You love to work with people. You love to work with your hands. You get a great deal of satisfaction from performing quick, magic-trick treatments. Your mastery of surgical skill is immensely rewarding. It is impressive. In fact that's why you have a growing practice. Your patients are impressed too. They like to see fast results.

Now you see it. Now you don't. Presto!

There are physicians who are happy working for eight-hour wages but the gravitational pull of a profitable specialty was overwhelming. You will fight like a mongoose to protect the independence, power, and prestige your profession has earned you.

Administrator

You administer a $50 million budget with a bureaucracy forced on you by regulation and tradition. Neither you, your board of directors, nor your medical staff speaks in public about the business of medicine. People want to believe hospitals are charitable, social service agencies. It is best to leave well enough alone. But, in your town of 100,000 people, 140 million health care dollars change hands each year. It is big business. When you are running at 50 percent capacity as you are today, 130 terribly ill patients depend on you every day. That adds up to 47,450 patient days per year. Those patients are reason enough to keep your institution alive.

You miss the golden years. Those days of glory were the ones before October 1, 1983. On that date the federal government changed the health care rules. Diagnostic Related Groups (DRGs) were introduced. In the old days hospitals were guaranteed a profit. The government, insurers, and patients paid whatever they were charged. It was a priceless cost-plus system. The DRGs set the price in advance. Overspending now has a consequence.

For instance, a craniotomy pays the hospital $9,970.40 whether the patient is hospitalized for five days or five months. It pays the same whether you provide excellent service or poor service. The secure income promised by old-fashioned medicine was one reason you worked for a master's degree in public health. DRG payments place your paycheck at risk.

When you were in school, the wholesale hospitalization of America was a given. It was more important for a hospital administrator to know about epidemiology than the fundamental business disciplines of marketing and finance. Bigger was better. Sick people were best cared for in a hospital. Cadillac medicine and surgical services were pronounced a birthright by President Lyndon B. Johnson. Both houses of congress approved.

The 1960s health care model spawned awesome construction projects. You built a career milestone on that model by securing $18 million on the bond market. The money built a new wing for more beds, added the technology your community demanded, and purchased the finest data processing hardware available. You were a hero.

Less than four years later, the data processing system is hopelessly inadequate. The technology is dated. The wing is empty.

On any given day the combination of DRGs and same day surgery technology keeps half of your city's hospital beds empty. Where are all the sick people? Patients used to spend weeks recovering. Now even heart catheterization patients are out in an afternoon.

Your hospital is the largest employer in the county. The competing hospital is third. Together you are the spinal cord in your local economy's backbone. Labor accounts for almost half of your budget. Hospital services require the skills of bright people.

Bright people who have spent their hard-earned dollars on expensive educations expect to be paid well. Salaries and benefits average more than $30 thousand per year per employee and there are still unionization efforts.

Employees regularly complain about their pay, many with good reason.

Graduate degree nurses make less money per hour than clerks at the local grocery store. Your wife, a critical care registered nurse, saw the light and started a catering business. Demands for higher wages are justified but money is tight. Quick corrections are impossible.

Plant operations, food, drugs, supplies, interest, and insurance account for another third of your operating expenses. The hospital's $500,000 insurance premium, a 20 percent increase over the previous year, knocked the wind out of you. Of course, it wasn't as bad as last year's 40 percent increase, or the 35 percent hit you took the year before. Good thing the hospital hasn't had any unfavorable judgments against it.

Finally, the cost of caring for others is a killer. Charity care, bad debt, and the negotiated charge reductions you gave to Blue Cross/Blue Shield in the hopes of increased volume oxidize your bottom line. The largest health care customers on earth, Medicare and Medicaid, deduct 20 cents of every dollar you bill prior to payment.

Few business ventures can hope to stay in business when customers get first-rate service by paying deeply discounted charges. On the other hand, the government is one customer who buys services without asking for so much as a warranty.

Your hospital gives away food, shelter, and medication to every man, woman, and child who is able to find his or her way into your building and ask for it. Every patient is entitled, regardless.

Last year a 45-year-old lifetime chain smoker played off the sympathy of the press. She appealed to her congressman and won $235,000 for a heart and lung transplant. Six months later she died of cirrhosis.

Fiduciary responsibility is part of managing a hospital. It cannot be taken lightly. You must niche the market with your services or you and your Board of Directors will default on massive loans. Over 900 employees would be without jobs.

Up until 1983 the more money you spent the more money you made. You never wanted or needed to know which services were cash cows and which were dogs as long as the hospital earned a profit. Now you know exactly what each service line costs to deliver.

Obstetrical services confound you. Poorly educated, expectant mothers who live in near poverty are prime candidates for low birth weight, handicapped babies. Tobacco, alcohol, and drug use is commonplace. Poor nutrition is a way of life. A rags-to-riches lawsuit tempts them.

Six of your eight obstetricians grew weary of the 24-hour-a-day call. The constant stream of threatened lawsuits wore them out. They quit delivering.

Hopefully, the obstetrics refresher course your emergency room doctors took will be enough to see you and the new moms through. Deliveries will have to be done without the help of a specialist.

That kind of problem is a minor detail for Medicaid, health maintenance organizations, and other insurers. Your hospital is expected to deliver comprehensive care to each and every patient. If you can't deliver, they will take all their business elsewhere.

Their focus is on money so you must focus on money, too. Their policy payouts must be whittled down so you carve out your charges. Any miscalculation in judgment, arithmetic, or politics is fraught with financial risk.

In the good old days you could shift the cost of care from people who had no insurance coverage to those who did. It was an approved solution. Cost shifting is no longer acceptable. Everyone claims the high moral ground on the health care battlefield until they have to pay for it. Like it or not, a patient's ability to pay for services rendered is a deciding factor in every patient's treatment plan. Visions of immortality built fixed costs into your medical center's operation. Operations have to produce the cash to cover those dreams.

There is one black hole and one cash flow sunbeam in the financial performance for your institution. Health promotion is a loser; surgical procedures are profitable.

The 25 heart, 30 back, and 40 gynecological surgeries your doctors will do this month will net your hospital more than the $50,000 you banked with your award-winning, home-grown health promotion venture HEALTH HABIT. As a bonus, surgical procedures generate the patient volume you need to support your ancillary service departments. The lab, dietary, respiratory therapy, physical therapy, and occupational therapy thrive when surgeries are up.

The nostalgia you feel for health promotion remains, but it is impractical to pursue. The government insists on paying for medical and surgical treatment. Your hospital stays in business by accommodating market demand. Last week the hospital joint-ventured a lobby restaurant with McDonald's.

REFERENCES

1. Commission on Professional and Hospital Activities. *International Classification of Diseases,* 9th Revision, Clinical Modification. Ann Arbor, MI: Edwards Brothers, Inc., 1978.

2. American Psychiatric Association. *Diagnostic and Statistical Manual of Mental Disorders,* 3rd ed. Washington, DC: GPO, 1978.

5

TWENTY-TWO HOURS AND 45 MINUTES—MARCH 1990

Act One

County hospital—6:00 p.m.

Beeeeeeeeeep!

"Dr. Jobe, Medic 1 is five minutes out with a 27-year-old female victim of a two-car MVA. No seat belt. Blood pressure is 60/40. Pulse 140. Respirations 24 and labored. They have a 3-year-old child on board. He doesn't appear to be injured. Fire fighters and paramedics are at the scene trying to extricate the driver in the other car."

Ten people crashed into the hallway—two respiratory therapists, an X-ray technician, a lab technician, a recording clerk, two nurses, and a nursing supervisor. Our hospital controller told me yesterday, "Your team costs me $220 an hour, plus benefits."

I told him, "We are a bargain. Wait until you need us sometime."

"Medic 1. This is Dr. Jobe. What is your patient's status and ETA?"

"Medic 1 here. Patient status is the same. Barely palpable BP, 60/40. Pulse 150. Shallow labored respirations. Patient was the driver in a head-on collision. She hit the steering wheel. There are contusions on her chest and abdomen. I'm not getting good breath sounds in her left chest. Her child was strapped into a car seat. He's upset. No injuries visible. ETA one minute."

"Julie. We need a chest tube tray set up and two large-bore IVs with normal saline. Lay the MAST trousers out. I'll need respiratory therapy to support ventilation with a bag mask and 100 percent O_2. Be ready for intubation. We'll have to check arterial blood gases immediately. I want a nasogastric tube and a Foley catheter."

A hemorrhaging patient means an AIDS risk. Gowned, gloved, and goggled, we looked like an Environmental Protection Agency SWAT team.

"Alert the operating room," I said. "Find the on-call surgeon. Give him a patient report. We'll need a chest X-ray right away."

Patients who narrowly escape death often have out-of-body experiences. I have an out-of-body experience every time a trauma patient rolls into my emergency room. I learned to leave my body during my three years of residency. I can view any scene with complete detachment. It is the best way to deal with this job.

Last week a friend of mine came in with multiple gunshot wounds. He had been hit 12 times by 9mm bullets. Hot lead crushed his left side. He looked like he fell 300 feet into a rock bed of barbed wire. A crazy transient sauntered up to him in his yard and opened fire.

Twelve hours of surgery saved his life. He was off the ventilator, fighting an infection, and looking down the gun barrel of at least four more major surgeries. But he was over the hump. Thank God his insurance will protect him from the costs of trauma care.

Flashing lights and sirens screamed around the corner of a hospital entrance. Don't screw up, I told myself.

"Ambulance here," said Julie Revson. The rig shut down its light show and sound system. "Trauma room's set up."

Julie is a good nurse. She has been a good nurse for 20 years. Time enough for strawberry blonde hair to drift into snow white. Her kind of nursing experience is next to impossible to find. Too many good nurses leave direct patient care to advance their careers. More dignity. More respect. More money. Fewer hassles. A lower risk for AIDS. Who can blame them?

The patient's distended belly cut me off from the ether of emotion. A seat belt could have saved her. "Have the social worker call her family. Is her kid OK?"

"OK. Yeah."

A paramedic held a mask over her face. He forced oxygen and life into her.

I gave orders to a nurse and a paramedic. "Start two large bore IVs. One in each arm. Dump in as much saline as you can. Draw blood for CBC, bleeding parameters. Type and cross for eight units fresh whole blood. Get the lab moving, STAT. I want the RT to put in a #8 endotracheal tube. See if we can't ventilate her better. I need a 16-gauge, 2½-inch needle, and syringe."

Good trauma care is fast. It's intelligent instinct.

The sound I heard with my stethoscope confirmed the paramedic's diagnosis. Breathing was decreased on the left side. That meant a collapsed lung until proven otherwise. Time to get down to business. I hate shoving big needles into people, but—here goes.

"You're going to feel a needle stick on your left side. Sorry." Three inches below the left armpit, just above the rib...PUNCH.

The needle pierced her chest. It slid into the space that usually is filled with a lung. Air gushed through the syringe. It relieved the pressure. The lung re-expanded. My right ear listened to another part of our treatment team.

"Patient intubated." We were in sync. "I can ventilate better."

"Inflate the MAST suit." I rolled off orders. "We need that chest X-ray. I'm putting in the chest tube. I want a Foley catheter inserted. Check the urine for blood. Recheck the BP. Put the patient on the cardiac monitor."

What a rush. I was backstroking in my element. This is what I'd trained to do. There weren't 10 other people in 50 square miles who could do this work.

"IVs are running. Wide open."

"MAST suit up."

"BP 75/40. Better."

Sweat fell from my brow. I stared at the drop on my hand. Rock steady. Hope I never get Parkinson's disease. Two more directives. "Cut away her clothes. Set up for a chest tube."

My first needle was out of her chest. I used another to inject a local anesthetic. My one-inch incision made her flinch.

"Mrs. Jameson," I apologized. "I know this hurts. I'm sorry. It'll be over in a second."

POP. What a rude sound.

The hemostat pops air into her chest. I pushed a ½-inch diameter, two-foot long tube halfway into the chest and attached it to suction. Blood and air were sucked out. The lung was supposed to expand.

"Take a deep breath," I told her. "Cough. Take a deep breath," I repeated, "you need oxygen."

I was talking to the wrong person. She couldn't breathe now if she had to. Respiratory therapy was breathing for her.

"She looks better," an optimist said.

"Her BP won't come up."

There is a life and death struggle on my table, in my hands. The only obvious signs of trauma are bruises on her chest and belly. Her belly is blowing up. She's bleeding. I'm not helping.

"Call the OR. Tell them we're not making progress," I ordered. "She'll need an exploratory. She's got to be belly bleeding. Let's get her out of here."

"I want my mommy! I want my mommy!"

I wanted to throw up. Maybe I should have been a chiropractor like my father. Spinal adjustments are never like this.

"Tommy. Tommy. Listen to me, Tommy," I said as I lifted him into a physical assessment hug. "Your mommy is going to be OK," I assured him. "She has an 'oooowee.' We're making it better. She's going to be fine," I lied.

Emergency department—6:40 p.m.

"Ambulance three minutes out, 41-year-old male," Julie said. "Confused. Small scalp laceration. Otherwise stable. BP 120/84. Pulse 82. Respirations, 16. Paramedics say he reeks of ETOH. Sounds like a drunk with a bump on his head." Julie paused. "Drunks always come out smelling like a rose, a Wild Irish Rose."

Last month Julie's 18-year-old son, an only child, was killed when a drunk driver hit him and his brand new mountain bike. The guy left him to die in a drainage ditch by the side of the road. The drunk came to a stop after hitting a 20-mile-an-hour speed limit sign two miles down the road. The drunk was so sloppy he couldn't understand why he was being arrested. He didn't know he'd hit anything, including the sign.

"Put him in trauma room 3," I said. "Ask Nadine to take Tommy to the cafeteria for a chocolate milk shake until his dad gets here. Would you like that Tommy?"

"I wanna stay with you."

"I know you do," I said. "I want to stay with you, too. But I have to go to work now. Other people need my help."

I took the microphone. "Medic 1. This is County Hospital. Tell me about this guy."

"ETA one minute," Perry answered. "He's a 41-year-old white male. Crossed a center line. Nailed the mother and son we just sent in. He got trapped in his car. Well, actually he wasn't trapped; he was too drunk to scramble out the window. The firemen used their Jaws of Life for practice. They ripped the car apart."

"Vitals are stable," Perry reported. "He stinks of sour mash whiskey. I'll bet three to one his blood alcohol is more than .30. Anyone want to bet?"

"Can it Perry."

"I found one small laceration above his right ear. We went through protocol. He's moving everything symmetrically to pain. We put a cervical collar on. Got him on the backboard. Sandbagged his head and started a large bore IV line with saline. Gave him an amp of D-50-W and two milligrams of Narcan. No change. How about five-to-one odds?"

I heard them cut off the siren. I didn't take his odds. The brief silence triggered my meat wagon memories.

When I was growing up ambulances were called meat wagons. They had one protocol: scoop up the patient, throw him in the rear of a red and white station wagon and race to a hospital.

When they arrived, everyone waited for a doctor to show up. The doc eventually rolled in wearing his civvies. He'd treat with whoever he could find to help. More than once it was a clerk or a housekeeper. The nurses were smart enough to scatter.

Unrehearsed chaos ruled. No one knew who to pity, the patient or the poor ophthalmologist who was taking his mandated weekend emergency room call. The guy hadn't used a stethoscope in 15 years. The last time he'd seen trauma was on the coast of Normandy.

The horror stories finally became too big to hide.

On prom night, 1978, six graduating seniors riding in a proud father's Cadillac were hit by a train. The Chief of Staff's daughter died at the hospital before the dermatologist on call for the emergency room could see past her acne and treat her ruptured spleen. The next weekend County Hospital had 24-hour-a-day coverage in the ER.

It is depressing to be old enough to see history repeat itself. Funding cuts have shut down six hospitals in our region during the past two years. Community ambulance companies went broke. Nine years of emergency medical services progress went into the dumpster.

Last weekend the Cat's Eye volunteer fire department brought a motor vehicle accident (MVA) victim in with a red and white Bronco. Their efforts were heroic, but the woman was gone when she got here. A year ago front-line drugs, proper equipment, and trained paraprofessionals would have made her an easy save. Those days are gone until some bigwig politician loses a wife or child to cost savings.

A gurney with the drunk rolled by me and into Room 3. I followed it.

"Mr. Pitstick," I said. "Can you hear me Mr. Pitstick? Mr. Pitstick, can you hear me? Wake up." I pinched his arm to get a response. I pinched harder.

Mr. Pitstick brushed my hand away. Probably thought I was a fly.

"Quit that!" he crabbed. He tried to go back to sleep. No deal. I was going to wake him up. I used my fingernails.

"Goddamn it! Quit that."

"Wake up, Mr. Pitstick," I said. "You are in the hospital."

"Where?"

"In the hospital," I said. "You've had an accident."

"What the hell?" he slurred. "Where's my car? I didn't bang up my car, did I?"

Perry whispered, "You wanna take my odds now? I'll give you six to one."

"I only bet through my bookie." Definitely more than a .30 blood alcohol. "Totaled," I answered, "cut to pieces by the fire department."

"Aw, shit."

Almost in spite of myself I began a head to toe obsessive-compulsive check. There was only a two percent possibility something was really wrong. But, that's what I get paid to do.

My dad always told me, "When you've got a job to do, do it well." And I do.

My attitude never fails me. This is the guy who will sue me, the nurses, the hospital, the ambulance company and win. No time for slipshod medicine.

"Mr. Pitstick," I said. "Wake up."

"What?" he asked again. "Where am I?"

"You're in the hospital. You've been in an accident."

I continued the examination process out of habit. I've done it 1,000 times. Practice makes perfect if the practice is perfect. Step by step.

Head. Three centimeter laceration above the right ear. Eyes. Pupils round. Reactive to light. Normal extraocular movement. Normal intraocular examination. Fundi discs and vessels. Ears. Normal tympanic membrane. No battle signs. Nose. No deviation. Normal airflow.

Julie worked her way through the trauma flow check-off sheet. She gave me aural and graphic vital signs.

"Anything on physical?" she asked.

"A cut above the right ear. Altered sensorium. I can't assess his neck until we take some cross table X-rays." I continued, "A bruise on his chest. Probably from the steering wheel. We need lab for CBC, urinalysis, blood alcohol, and X-rays for his chest and C-spine. We need an EKG, too."

Perry butted in, "You going to CAT scan this guy's head? Odds are going up. I'm giving seven-to-one."

"You got an inside tip?"

"State Patrol just showed up," he said. "This is Mr. Pitstick's fifth DWI and second major wreck in four months. His license is suspended. He has no insurance. I'm giving you the only chance you've got to make some money on this one. Seven-to-one going once. Going twice."

"Chill out."

Perry ducked behind a screen. Good move. We had the rest of the night to work together.

Yeah. I had to CT scan his head. CT scans are state-of-the-art care. Mr. Pitstick's lawyer would point out that fact if I neglected to do one. I would be likened to a doctor who forgets to take a pulse when he's checking for a heartbeat.

With the black and white Brownie prints our radiology department processed 10 years ago, this problem would've never come up. Today CT scans turn out radiographic Monets.

Painters and radiologists have the same skills. They create beautiful images. They capture the landscape on first-rate canvas. Their pictures are beautiful. They are expensive. Everyone wants to own an original even if it costs a fortune.

Good CT head scans run $600 apiece without a frame.

I claim a 95 percent level of confidence with my clinical diagnostic skills. A 95 percent level of confidence is terrific for a two dollar bet. It is worthless for diagnosing patients.

If one out of 20 of my patients leaves this ER with a wrong judgment call, I'm out my job and everything I own in life. To cover my rear end, I add science. Science gets the odds down to 100-to-one.

Even at those odds, 30 of my 3,000 annual patients are potential lawsuits. Mr. Pitstick's lab tests, X-rays, and CT scans will set the hospital back $1,000. Not taking a scan could set us back millions.

Emergency department—7:00 p.m.

"Matthew. We've got a dead baby in room 4." Julie was looking at the floor. "It's Mr. Richards."

"Let me guess," I said. "Their baby fell down the steps."

"Yep."

"Damn. Call the cops. See if we can put him in jail this time. I'll go see the family."

I examined the tiny corpse. I called the county coroner. Then I went to the private conference room. I'd met Mr. Richards last year after his five-year-old daughter supposedly fell down the steps. She rolled in DOA, too.

"Hello, doctor. Is he going to be all right?" Richards asked with indifference. The same indifference he'd used to inquire about his daughter.

"I'm afraid not," I said. "Your son was dead when he arrived."

"Oh, no." Vacant emotion. "I can't believe it." That's what he said in April.

"How did this happen?" I probed for an honest answer.

"He was playing with his ball on the steps and he fell down."

He's not even going to bother to make up a different story. "When did it happen?" I inquired.

"Just afer lunch," he answered. "I put him down for a nap and went to the neighbor's to watch the ball game."

"I went in to kiss him when I got home from work at four o'clock," said Mrs. Richards. "He was sound asleep. This is terrible," she observed.

"Yeah. This is terrible."

It is terrible. The police were standing outside.

"Can we go home now?" they asked. "There's nothing else we can do."

"The police have some questions for you to answer," I said. "It will only take a little time." Or, with luck, life without parole.

I walked away. A bulletin board sign caught my eye. Printed in large block black letters the nursing station message read, WE DO OUR BEST TO KEEP THIS ROOM NEAT AND TIDY. IF SOMEONE BEFORE YOU HAS LEFT A MESS, PLEASE LET US KNOW.

Emergency department—7:15 p.m.

"Code 4. Room 226. Code 4. Room 226. Code 4. Room 226." What the paging system really means to say is, "Someone is trying to die in Room 226. Someone is trying to die in Room 226. Someone is trying to die in Room 226."

Hospital administration doesn't like to have patients dying in our hospital. High mortality statistics are frowned upon by the American Association of Retired Persons, the government's Health Care Financing Administration, and the press. We all work extra hard to keep patients alive until they leave.

Rumor has it that if patients die on their way out the door, the nurses are supposed to turn them around to make it look like they were coming in.

I ran out past a teenage girl, a derelict who had thrown up on himself and our carpet, and a druggie who looked like he wanted a new prescription for Percodan. "Julie. Get the CT scan and tell the patients what's happening. I'll be back as soon as I can."

I wonder what the patients think when they see a doctor running away from them. I've never asked. A little old lady shouted a complaint at me, "How long do I have to wait to see a doctor around here? My bowels haven't moved for seven days. I can't stand it another minute."

Our code team falls in like a marine platoon at reveille. We have spent hours together in drill.

When a Code is called we round up our $100,000 worth of equipment, our $275,000 in talent, and head for the specified room. Network sports should sponsor code team competition. Even then we would be a shamefully affordable franchise.

I always ache for the coded patient's roommate. He is asleep, recuperating from an appendectomy and gaining strength. Suddenly a cult experience breaks loose at his bedside.

Strange faces run into his room. They surround his buddy. They pounce on him. He watches. He listens in horror. Who are these people? Is this happening? Could I be next if I'm not careful?

"Check the airway and pulse," I ordered. "I want a summary from the patient's nurse. Call the private doc."

"Airway clear. No spontaneous respiratory movement."

"Barely palpable femoral pulse. Slow. Maybe 50."

I recited my lines, "Ventilate him with a bag mask. Intubate when ready. Give him one milligram of Atropine intravenously." My team's Pavlovian response kicks in.

"Atropine given."

"Listen for bilateral breath sounds," I commanded.

"Boy! It's tough ventilating this guy." Sam, the respiratory therapist, was already sweating like a pig. "His lungs are like ham hocks in a pot of split pea soup."

"BP 90/60. Pulse up to 70."

"Cardiac monitor on. Here's a strip." I looked at the heart rhythm on a piece of graph paper. His electrical system was intact. His heart was pumping.

"It's a respiratory arrest," I announced. "Let's intubate." The sword swallower circus act. It's one of the best tricks they taught me in med school.

I slid the six-inch blade over the tongue and down the throat until I could see vocal cords.

"Suction."

We sucked out the sputum.

"Tube."

I slid Excalibur through his cords.

"Inflate." Janie put five cubic centimeters of air in the side port, inflated the bulb, and made a fit. Whoever invented this thing was a wizard.

"Bag him." When in doubt give an order, ask a question. "Someone listening to both lungs for breath sounds?"

"No breath sounds."

When apprehensive, give another order. "Listen to the stomach."

"The tube is in the esophagus," Jan said. "You're blowing air into the stomach."

When embarrassed, give two commands. "Deflate the tube. Bag him."

Sam put the mask over the patient's mouth and nose. "I can't get a good seal for pressures. Boy, is he stiff."

A pruned face, barreled chest, and nicotine-tattooed fingertips are dead giveaways of a lifetime smoker. Today was the day he'd been working for.

"Pulse back to 50. I can't get a blood pressure."

No oxygen. His heart was stopping.

When in trouble lead with two orders. "Intubating again. Suction. Tube."

"Inflate it. Ventilate him." Supreme confidence. Two orders and a question. "Breath sounds?"

"Loud and clear. Bilaterally good. Way to go!"

"How much time did we take?"

Sarah, today's code reporter, perked up. "One minute and 12 seconds from arrival."

"Seemed slow," I said. Our huddle was breaking up. Everyone was standing around trying to catch an emotion.

The roommate stared. Dumbfounded. He'd caught his feelings with his diaphragm. They knocked the wind out of him.

"Hyperventilate him," I said. "We need blood gases to see where we are."

"BP 95/70. Pulse is up to 70."

"Tell respiratory therapy and ICU we need a ventilator set up. Who can tell me about this guy?" I asked.

"He's my patient." Christie, a newly licensed nurse with sparkles still in her eyes, stepped forward. She held the patient's chart. It was three inches thick. "I've had him before," Christie said. "He is Dr. Smoleroff's patient. The doctor is on his way in. Mr. Taylor is a 56-year-old male with an 88-pack-year history of smoking."

Hmmmm. Let's see, I calculated. That is two packs per day for 44 years or three packs per day for nearly 30 years.

"He's had a morning cough for as long as he can remember. Lots of clear whitish sputum. By the way, this comes from his wife. The patient denies everything."

"The patient always does."

"He refused an admission to ICU," she continued. "Said he couldn't afford $1,000 a day."

"He's going to get billed for $1,000 a minute," someone joked. No one laughed.

"I walked in and found him gasping," said Christie. "I should have been with him but I've got seven other sick patients. I feel terrible."

You feel terrible, I thought, look at Mr. Taylor.

Blood gases showed low oxygen and high CO_2. The chest X-ray exposed massive quantities of fluid in his lungs. The endotracheal tube was in its proper position. No pneumothorax. Severe respiratory failure.

We had forced breath into him. Now he had no choice. We were going to breathe for him whether he wanted to or not.

I remember the panicky feeling I had one time as a kid when I choked on a piece of apple at the dinner table. I was scared to death. My dad hit me on the back and it was over. This guy had lived with that fear for three days. If only Mr. Taylor could enjoy such a simple solution.

"Repeat blood gases in 20 minutes to confirm improvement," I ordered. "Let's move him to ICU. Get him on a ventilator so RT can quit bagging him."

"Let's go," said Sarah. She was in a hurry to get back to the work she had dropped for the code. "I've got four more enemas to give tonight before I eat dinner."

Nurses hate enemas.

In my family, anyone who got sick got an enema. No questions asked. Right or wrong I learned it didn't pay to be sick. Whenever I get sick I don't dwell on it. I think about being well.

Emergency department—8:00 p.m.

Sharon, an ace LPN, was waiting for me. "There's a guy in Room 1 with a problem pee pee," she said. "Poooor guy. He tried to cop a feel. I karate chopped him and told him it was probably too BIG a problem for me to HANDLE."

"Thanks a lot." I guessed gonorrhea.

"Hi ya, Doc." I was impressed. Spiked hair, a safety pin earring, and a studded "David Lee Roth World Tour" jacket.

"What seems to be the problem?"

"Well you know how it is. I was getting some action last weekend," he explained. "I got a little something extra from a cherry tomato." Why do guys refer to their women as if they were fresh produce?

"You want to see my tool?" he grinned. "I tried to show it to the nurse, but she was cold. She walked out! Can't you teach them bitches a few manners?"

I bit my tongue. "We work pretty hard around here on courtesy," I said. "I'll speak with her about it. Please accept my apologies."

"That's OK. But I'd appreciate it if you would kick her ass for me. Maybe write her up."

"I doubt that I'll do that. Let's have a look." He dropped his jeans. His underwear was a mess. A science project.

"What do you think, Doc? It hurts like a mother when I piss. I thought it would go away but it never did."

We are going to have to amputate, I thought. "You've got the 'clap,'" I said.

"Ain't that a son of a bitch?" He beamed, "I've put my hamburger between a bunch of buns lately. I should have known I would get clapped sometime."

It's not applause, my friend. "You ought to use condoms next time."

"A rubber? Man, you gotta be kidding."

"You need the 'big one,' " I said.
"What?"
"The 'big needle.' "
He paled. "What's the 'big needle'?"
"Two point four million units of penicillin in each cheek."
"Sounds like it hurts," he said in falsetto.
"Hurts like a son of a bitch." Pills would work just as well, but pills don't teach the same lesson. I went back to my office, caught my breath, and saw the afternoon paper on my desk.

A cub reporter had beaten the coroner to the scene of an accident. Color picture. Page one. One ruined Harley Hog. One head in a helmet. The article read

DOCTOR KILLED

Dr. William Phillips, a prominent local physician, was fatally injured when he lost control of the motorcycle he was riding.

No, no, no, no. They got the story wrong. Bill lost control on cocaine and Quaaludes a year ago. I admitted him last week for an overdose of barbiturates. I couldn't convince him to enter treatment. What a waste.

He would have been 42. His third wife was packing her bags to leave. She couldn't stand his drinking anymore. He'd lost his practice. He was going to lose his privilege to practice. He couldn't make eye contact with anyone. He'd lost touch with everyone.

It looked to me as though he died from embarrassment. Bill was probably another undetected suicide.

Emergency department—9:30 p.m.

"Dr. Jobe," the intercom insisted, "we've got patients waiting."
"Sorry. I was looking at the newspaper."
"We're sorry too, doctor."
Julie handed me the next chart. A doozie. It's not even a full moon tonight!

I sutured the six-inch long slash along the patient's jaw and chuckled. "Good thing you didn't breathe on your camp fire. You'd have lit up like a bottle of 151."

He laughed. "It's cold out there. A shot of brandy now and then keeps me warm. There's a flask in my jacket if you want a toot."

I laughed with him. I used to get upset, rant, rave, and lecture. It finally dawned on me. No one was listening. Life is easier if you don't worry.

This guy was chopping branches off a 200-year-old live cedar tree for a Cub Scout marshmallow roast when the head popped off his double bit and hit him in the face.

"Why me, Doc?" he asked.

Emergency department—10:25 p.m.

"Dr. Jobe, Mrs. Pitstick's here."

I walked into the waiting room, anger intact. Someone was going to be held responsible.

The room was full. I scanned the couches for the accomplice. A young couple. My favorite hypochondriac transvestite, Billy. An old man. A mother with four bug-eyed children cowering in the corner. A man.

Where is she? I scanned the room again. This was going to be a long night.

"Mrs. Pitstick."

"Yes," she sobbed, holding onto her kids for support.

"I'm sure you know your husband was in an accident. He's going to be OK."

"I'm sorry. I'm so sorry. I'm sorry." Tears poured down her face.

I brought her and her children back into the examination room.

Something about her was familiar. I had to ask, "Do I know you?"

She searched my face, more for reassurance than recognition. "I don't think so."

"Did you ever live in Centerville, Ohio?" I asked.

"I grew up there," she said. "Matthew?"

"Joanie? Oh, Joanie." We embraced. "I'm so sorry."

Life had ravaged her. I would never have known her. Joanie was the kid sister of my senior class prom date, Ellen Ipiotis, a blonde cheerleader. I wanted to ask, "How's Ellen?" but I didn't.

I had tried to forget all about her and her family. I remember her father always had a 16-ounce tumbler of Scotch in his hand. Her mother slept on the couch in the afternoon. I'd heard her older brother died of cirrhosis in his late 20s. Joanie had married a man just like her father.

Joanie's three boys may already be alcoholics and they probably don't know it. The only way to keep them well would be to keep them away from drugs and alcohol.

"Joanie," I said, "I'm going to get you some help. We'll get a counselor down here right away. Give me a call tomorrow. Will you do that?"

"Yes. God. I am so sorry," she cried. Her kids were crying. I was starting to cry.

"I'll be back in a bit," I said, knowing I wouldn't.

"Julie, get the chemical dependency liaison down here. She's going to need help. Maybe we can get Mr. Pitstick into detox and treatment tonight. Maybe he can begin his recovery."

"Do you know her?" Julie asked.

"A long time ago."

"There's a granny nursing a broken hip in Room 3. A severe running nose is in Room 1."

Emergency department—11:30 p.m.

I walked into the examination room. Teenage parents with twins. Dual diarrhea.

There was a time when I treated these families free of charge. Honestly, they don't have enough to keep their kids fed. I found out after I had sent them on their way, many of them went to the ER across town.

A lady with 12 kids explained the mystery to me. "If it doesn't cost nothin', it's not worth nothin'."

One night a physician called in to say he was sending me a 13-year-old girl. She had fallen. Her elbow hurt. Her family was very poor. Could I help them out?

Sure.

I gave Cindy a thorough examination. She had full range of motion. She had a little pain in her elbow. I told her parents it was unlikely that anything was wrong. Since I hadn't done too much I said we could tear up the chart and I did. I told them to go see their regular doctor in two weeks. Her parents took Cindy to their doctor on schedule.

Their doctor took an office X-ray of her elbow. By using poor technique, dated equipment, and too much radiation, he managed to take a picture of little Cindy's entire arm. Her humerus was hairline fractured at the shoulder. Her pain had been referred to her elbow.

The break was healing well. It required no treatment. My initial diagnosis was wrong. An attorney told them to sue.

I had no documentation. No chart. I went to their house.

My plea for mercy succeeded. I learned my lesson.

Now I document everything. I charge everyone something. They value my opinion. I appreciate their payment.

When I came out of my parent conference, Julie looked happy. "Tommy's mother just got out of surgery. They stopped the bleeding. Her blood pressure is stabilizing."

"Great!" I applauded. "The OR does good work."

"Her spleen was pulverized. They had to remove it. She got to keep everything else—her lacerated liver, bruised kidney, and the bowel wall. She won't need a colostomy."

Now she needed time and good luck. Tommy needed good luck. So did Joanie.

Emergency department—11:45 p.m.

"What seems to be the problem here?" I asked as I reached for the newborn babe.

"Angela got that growth on her head two weeks ago," her mother told me. She pointed out the lump. "Our pediatrician looked at her. She sent us to a neurosurgeon."

"What did he say?"

"She is thinking about surgery."

"What brought you in tonight?" I asked as I washed the tumor.

"Our cat was licking it," she explained. "I was afraid it might get infected."

I smelled cinnamon. I washed the hairy growth again. I sniffed. Cinnamon. "Ma'am," I said in my "Sergeant Joe Friday" voice, "Angela has a piece of Halloween candy stuck to her head. I can fix her up."

Emergency department—12:11 a.m.

I reviewed the last three cases to strengthen my memory for the charting process that would have to wait until morning. One sore throat. Probably strep. One pelvic infection. Probably gonorrhea. One rape victim.

I first saw this girl on my way to the code. When she saw me leave, humiliation overwhelmed her and she left, too. She thought everyone in the waiting room could see what had happened to her.

Her parents brought her back. They helped her find the strength to face me. The bruises, blood, and semen confirmed her story. Now I get to witness a court confrontation. The last time this happened I testified against a Hell's Angel.

I lived through a death threat and gave my testimony so the biker could do 90 days.

This time it would be a little easier. I had the rapist's DNA fingerprint from his sperm. Her charge would be 99 percent fact. Unless, of course, the court blamed her for being attractive.

Not guilty is an easy verdict for a competent defense attorney to get.

He would choose nine men and three women. Chances are, at least two of the women would be racked with guilt about the times when they were forced to have sex. Chances are, eight of the men had exploited a female at least once in their life. Chances are, all 12 would deny their own sexual experiences.

She was accusing her high school senior class president—a 4.0 honor society member who was captain of the football, basketball, and track teams. Nothing to it. He turned 18 yesterday.

Julie stuck her head in my office. "We've got an ambulance coming in with a 68-year-old male. Sounds as though he was a complete cardiac arrest in the field, resuscitated by none other than our own administrator and his wife."

"Boy! That's P.R.," I said. "Wait until the story hits the papers."

"The paramedics report him to be stable with a blood pressure of 130/77. Respirations, 16. Pulse, 84. Occasional PVCs. They have given him 75 milligrams of lidocaine. They want to know if you want any more. The patient is alert and talking. He appears to be in no distress at this time."

"I'll be right out. Tell them not to administer any more medication."

I thought of how David and Sarah must feel now. Whoever did mouth-to-mouth probably feels like puking.

I'd met Roy about a year and a half ago at a hospital administration barbecue. Roy and I thought the fresh strawberries were the high point of the picnic.

"Roy?" I asked. "What are you doing here at this time of night?"

"Well hello, Dr. Jobe," he said. "I'm not doing so good." He was telling the truth.

"I thought he was a goner," said Helen.

"Yeah. I heard." The entire family listened intently. Roy had two hands held in each of his. "It's a good thing you've got good neighbors, Roy," I said.

"Don't I know it."

He knew it.

I examined him. I drew the lab work. I told him it was great he didn't smoke. I sent him on his way to the ICU to monitor his rhythm. "I think you're going to be out of here in a couple of days, but I want to keep an eye on you."

His EKG appeared to rule out a heart attack. Most likely Roy had an electrical short. We can fix bad circuitry with a simple piece of space age hardware, $14,000 plus installation. If Roy could get an implantable defibrillator to jump start his heart, it could mean five more years of the good life for him.

"I'll keep both eyes on him," said Helen. "Roy always says we've been together 60 years. Thirty for him and 30 for me. He's not going to get away from me now."

Emergency department—1:10 a.m.

"There's a blue bloater in Room 1," said Trisha, the float nurse who agreed to cover Julie's exit.

"Another pair of ham hocks?" I asked.

"Yeah."

Blue bloaters differ from pink puffers. Both have a COLD—Chronic Obstructive Lung Disease. Bloaters with chronic bronchitis flounder in the bay of secretion.

Emphysemic pink puffers have destroyed so much healthy tissue, their lungs can't produce a puddle. If, by chance, a puddle appeared, they wouldn't be able to clear it.

I could hear my patient coughing, hacking, and swallowing hockers. I walked in with a friendly greeting, "Good morning, Mr. Martin."

He wiped his mouth with his handkerchief and stuffed it into his back pocket. He switched the soggy tissues to his left hand and reached out to shake my hand.

"What's the trouble, Mr. Martin?"

"You're the doctor," Mr. Martin said. "You tell me."

"What brought you to the hospital tonight?" I asked.

"My neighbor."

I can't help if I can't get through. Confiding in anyone goes against the grain of people who are used to telling their family and friends, "Take a hike. I'll do as I please."

"How can I help you?" I asked.
"That's what I came here to find out."
"Don't you feel well?"
"If I felt well," he coughed, "I wouldn't be here."
"Tell me about your cough," I suggested.
"Cough?" he asked. "Can't you cut with all this crap?"
"Mr. Martin," I said, "believe me, I would rather be at home in bed with a good book. You've got to help me so I can help you." Confrontation was the only answer this time.
"My cough began three days ago," he said. "It's hard to breathe, especially when I move around."
All right. Progress. "Are you coughing anything up?"
"No," he said. "Well...I always cough things up."
"Has the color or consistency of your sputum changed?"
"No," he answered. "Well...it's a little more greenish now."
"Do you feel like you have a temperature?"
"Everyone has a temperature."
Three steps forward, one step back. "Have you been feeling hot and cold, like you have a fever?"
"Well, yeah."
"Do you smoke?"
"No." The burn holes in his shirt and pants tattled.
"Have you ever smoked?" I asked.
"I used to."
"When did you quit?"
"Three days ago when my cough began," he said.
"How much do you normally smoke?" I asked. "Three to four packs a day?" Start high and let the patient bring it down.
"Yeah."
He surprised me. Sixty to 80 cigarettes per day. Five an hour, 16 hours a day. "Started when you were a kid?" I asked.
"Age nine. Camels," he said. "I smoke Carltons now. They're low-tar."
"Have you had a chest X-ray recently?" I asked.
"Never," he hacked. "X-rays are dangerous." He swallowed a greenie and gagged again. "Can't you give me a shot of penicillin and let me go home? I want to go home."
"Have you ever had your blood checked?"
"No."
"Mr. Martin," I said, "before I can help you I need a blood count, some sputum to examine under the microscope, and a chest X-ray. Do you want my help?"
"Yeah." He swallowed hard. "I'm afraid, Doc. I'm afraid I'm going to die."
"We'll do our best to keep you alive. That's a promise."

Emergency department—5:10 a.m.

The last couple of hours flew by. A ruptured ovarian cyst. Now in surgery.

A negative pregnancy screen at 3:00 a.m. She is probably back in bed asleep. Another case of strep throat. A two-car, one-motorcycle accident with five multiple trauma victims.

The world has another 23-year-old dirt bike quadriplegic to care for.

The last patient of the night was a young woman with a headache. She'd lost her Tylenol #3 prescription. She swore she would report me to the county medical society for not giving her narcotics.

Now to recall everything that was said and done. Completing 37 charts at five in the morning is enough to make me sick.

Act Two

The Solomons' bathroom—5:45 a.m.

Roy's crunching ribs came at me when I looked myself in the mirror. I could still feel the life force moving from my hands into Roy. I finished my shave. I flossed my teeth. I dressed and had breakfast.

I pulled the rubber band off my morning paper and read a headline. It had been a tough night for our ER.

MAN HELD IN DEATH OF
TWO-YEAR-OLD SON

I recognized the dad's name. He should have been put in the slammer last year. His lawyer used erratic hospital charting as a defense. At least he was in jail this morning. My next door neighbor and friend, the public defender, had a new client. I turned the page and another headline made me reel.

SMITH GETS 90 DAYS

Johnny Smith, aged 37, was placed on four years' probation and sentenced to 90 days in the county jail in connection with the March death of his 5-month-old daughter. Smith pleaded guilty to negligent homicide.

Smith told the court he was carrying his daughter down the stairs and fell. Her brother, Joey, 4 months old, died under similar circumstances on July 30, 1985.

Sirhan Sirhan would have been paroled long ago if he had killed his kids.

The physicians' parking lot was full of personality at 6:00 a.m. including the cardiac surgeon's Porsche, his physician assistant's Cherokee, the anesthesiologist's Audi, the orthopod's Corvette, and the chaplain's '63 slant six-cylinder Valiant. Business looks brisk.

The ER was a pit.

I picked up a few instruments at the foot of the empty gurney and put them on the desk.

"Long night?" I asked.

"You could say that," said Matthew.

"How's Roy?"

"I haven't had a chance to sit down since he came in," he said over a stack of charts. "No news is good news."

Charts. Pristine reports that tell the whole story and none of it. Drunken drivers are coded as trauma. Overdoses are respiratory arrests. Cancers are carcinomas. If charts were accurate they would read: Alcohol. Depression. Drugs. Tobacco.

"You and Sarah did a good job."

"Thanks."

Ruth and Joyce, two day-shift RNs, came in for report and began to clean up the mess. A restoration of sparkle and shine would take two hours minimum. A peculiar quiet fell over the department. Someone was about to speak their mind.

Trisha, a night shift RN, hadn't gone home yet from her 12-hour shift. She was talking to a young woman who had just flashed her Magic Kingdom Medicaid card. The nasty nickname our staff uses for the public assistance identification pass did fit the circumstance. This patient had used her card before.

Practice makes perfect.

Trisha and the card holder sat together at the free blood pressure check desk. She assessed the woman's chapped lips.

"What should I do about my lips?" she blistered. "They hurt like hell when I French kiss my man."

"I would use Vaseline or some sort of lip balm."

"Are you a doctor?" she asked indignantly.

"No," Trisha said.

"I came here to see a doctor."

"A doctor's office is cheaper," explained Trisha.

"I don't have time to wait in a doctor's office," the woman bitched, "that takes all day."

The woman bit off a piece of skin from her lower lip while she chewed on Trisha. "I've got Medicaid. Doctors don't cost nothin'."

"Your doctor costs someone something," Trisha informed her. "I'm probably paying for you."

The patient stormed out. She scolded, "You'll never see me here again. Not in this hospital!"

The staff applauded. The admitting clerk cheered, "I've wanted to say that for nine years!" Her mouth dropped when she saw me.

I walked away shaking my head. They missed our customer service mark by a mile but I couldn't find the wherewithal to reprimand them this morning. I had to go to a bioethics committee meeting.

I entered the meeting room thinking, society owes its people a fair exchange, not a free exchange. I braced myself with black coffee.

Dr. Schumaker, a neurologist, began the meeting. "Thank you all for coming." His Tennessee accent made everyone feel down home.

"Mr. and Mrs. Hahn have asked us for counsel," he said. "They want to review their options for a difficult decision."

This is the only committee meeting I attend with no absences. Six physicians, six nurses, two ministers, one nun, a lawyer, the district attorney, a psychologist, and I always clear our calendars to be here. I guess it's easier to participate in these decisions than to read about them under a happy-go-lucky headline in *USA Today*.

"Mr. Hahn, please give us an overview of the problem."

"I just want to say... first of all... I am thankful you are trying to help us." He was stumbling. So were the rest of us.

"I just got out of jail. I was in three years. My wife and me are trying to start over," Mr. Hahn said. "I got a good job washing dishes. Ruby cleans houses."

"We got four kids," Mrs. Hahn said. Her flower print dress was pressed and pretty. She gripped a rosary.

The confessions were over. The Hahns appeared to relax a bit. Their values, their position were respected. It looked to me like this was the first time in their lives this consideration had been extended to them.

"Two days ago we had a baby." Her voice cracked. Her eyes glistened. "Our baby is deformed."

As she spoke, I scanned my summary sheet. Her daughter was born hydrocephalic with a cleft palate, no ears, and esophageal atresia—no esophagus.

"She can't eat," Mrs. Hahn said. "We don't have no money." She could not continue.

A man in a tan, doubleknit leisure suit who I did not recognize opened his mouth. "I have offered to help the Hahns. Let us bow our heads for the Lord's prayer as we work to ensure this child's survival."

Ambushed. We bowed our heads. The Hahns' baby was being gypped out of the reasoned response I had promised her parents.

"Amen."

I wanted to adjourn the meeting. I waffled.

Mr. Hahn's voice was desperate. "I was just getting it together man. This'll put me in the joint again."

Dr. Schumaker stepped into an uncomfortable pause. "Mr. and Mrs. Hahn, as a physician I can tell you there are many things we can do to help you and your family. You are not alone." He explained every option. My headache was lifting.

The Hahns held hands and they listened.

"Your family resources will not have to be exhausted, Mr. Hahn," said the DA. "The State has resources for this kind of situation. We have a strong foster home system in our community." He took his time. He outlined a broad network of public and private human services.

"Our hospital will keep the baby until we find the best way to help," I said, sensing the hospital would be expected to pick up the tab.

"But my baby can't even take my milk," Mrs. Hahn said. "How will she live?"

"We will feed her the way we feed other patients who can't eat," I said. "It is easy to do." If I am to err, I choose to err with my peers.

"Can our baby be baptized?"

"I'll call Father Ritchie today," Sister Elizabeth gently assured them.

After an hour, we reached a consensus. The child would stay in the hospital until she could be placed in a home. She would be fed for however long she would live. If she fit her statistical profile, she'd hang on 30 days. The hospital would be out $30,000.

We watched the end of life roulette wheel spin to a stop. We had a winner. Last month the marble cut a comatosed junkie off antibiotics. He died of pneumonia in 48 hours.

Dr. Whiteman, our committee's psychologist, answered my $64,000 ethics question once. She said, "Life support systems are for the family, not the patient. Those machines help survivors come to grips with an impending loss. Some of us need more time than others. However much time money buys is spent."

She told me, "It's simple. People don't like to see other people die. It is better to have a committee decide when the time is right for a person to pass on. A committee's decision is less painful and less vulnerable to veto."

Four weeks ago, six months of family planning independent of our committee was destroyed in a moment. A lymphoma patient had chosen to die in a hospital bed. He could access all the pain medication he wanted. His wife and his doctor supported his wishes. A "Do Not Resuscitate" chart order was written.

The patient nearly expired on a Sunday night three days after his admission. His physician was out of town. Another internist stepped in. That doctor called a code and prolonged the purgatory of his death.

The patient's wife appealed to him. He rebuffed her. "I will have no part of murder." Nice soft touch.

The man died early the next day with his doctor and wife by his side. The internist's intervention cost the family $2,650 and another 24 hours of heartbreak.

I cannot honestly bring myself to believe God preferred a late Monday to an early Sunday homecoming.

Administration—8:00 a.m.

"Thanks, Rosie." She handed me the morning census report.

"You are welcome," said Rosie. "It's a good day for business."

"I hope so," I fretted.

"Say, do you know what is brown and black and looks good on a lawyer?"

"No. What?"

"A Doberman," chuckled Rosie. "I just love that joke."

I finished my morning reading, an editorial entitled, "The Dilemma of Access to Quality Medical Care in Rural Communities." Hospital journals suffer from terminal headlines.

Jack walked in with his mug of caffeine. "Look at these numbers," he said, "they're depressing."

Between his need to see columns of figures, and my need to see a big picture, we try to get one whole-brained look at the day.

"I heard you were a hero last night."

"No," I said. "Sarah was the hero. She told me what to do and I followed directions."

"Was it bad?"

"Ugly. I keep hearing Roy hit the floor. Let's talk about something else. How is the Mexican national in intensive care doing?" I asked.

"His bill is $173,000," Jack replied. "He's got another 45K to recovery."

"He's a miracle," I said. "When he rolled that '62 Ford pickup, he broke every bone in his body except the ones in his inner ear. We got to strut our stuff. Some skinflint will say we should have let him die. Did we ever find out where he was from?"

"Some no-name town in Mexico. No family. No friends. No nothing. He picked a great place to have a critical injury crash." Jack waved adios.

I am glad we can still afford to take care of the migrants who travel through town. It's the people who can afford to pay their debts and don't who get my goat.

Yesterday's bad debt story of the week took the cake. Patient No. 408321 had a triple bypass on Friday the 13th. He left town before he paid the surgeon. He mailed his doctor a note from Fiji saying he couldn't afford to pay his bill. I didn't believe it myself until I saw the palm tree postcard steri-stripped to the surgery schedule blackboard.

I heard a knock on my open door. I looked up to see our hospital marketing and sales force.

"Good morning," Tim said. "I've got some bad news for you. But I've got some good news for you, too."

"It's morning," I said. "Let's have it all."

"That gangland hit yesterday is the bad news and the good news. The guy who got gunned down was a benefits manager for the company I called on last week. He wasn't interested in our Employee Assistance Program."

Tim continued, "On Monday, he told me our program was against company policy. The company's owner called this morning to say they've changed their mind and I should come right over. Two hundred and forty employees!"

"Good job, Tim. That's a heck of a way to close a sale."

"I'll have them sign the bottom line today."

"Did you check on that Minnesota hospital?" I asked. "I was impressed with their plastic surgery financing program."

"I got an answering machine."

"You're kidding."

"I swear," he swore. "It said, 'Samaritan Hospital is closed. For information on billing call 434-1894.'"

"No."

"Yes!" said Tim. "I called the billing number. The guy who answered the phone sounded terrible."

"I bet. What did he say?"

"I asked him if Sheila Ring, their marketing director, was still employed. He said, 'No one works here anymore.' Can you imagine that?"

"I can today."

Tim was off. He left me to my thoughts.

Here I am running a $50 million a year service business. I've got one salesman. Some day Tim and I will figure out a way to sell hospital health services the way tobacco companies and breweries sell their products. Aggressively, competitively, effectively. No apologies.

Those guys promote their wares without shame. Management assumes the cost of sales and advertising, and promotions are 20 percent of their product's price tag.

If our promotion and sales costs were 20 percent of the patient's treatment, we'd be packed with patients. We'd have to hire Bartles and Jaymes to thank everyone for their support. Fat chance of that happening.

Our industry still labors under the illusion that persuasive communication is beneath its dignity. We haven't learned a thing from our court dates with the pterodactyls of the legal system.

At least we are finally using market research.

Two years ago we conducted our first public opinion survey. We wanted to know if employers were aware of any employee mental health, alcohol, and drug problems.

Tim interviewed 25 businesses in this town. None of their 12,546 employees had any personal problems. No alcoholism. No addiction. No depression.

Sad to say our hospital's personnel department was of the same opinion. Tim's insistence and an employee death changed a lot of minds about the need for and the benefits of counseling in the work site.

Brenda Watson's suicide came as a shock. She was the best social worker we had. Brenda was the tower of strength we leaned on. Craziness knows no holiday. She did herself in on Thanksgiving Day two years ago. One bullet to her brain.

We needed help in dealing with the stress her sudden death caused. The gospel according to John provided the answer. John was a new employee who sported a doctorate in psychology from Harvard.

The first thing John did at our debriefing was to place a box of Kleenex on the table. Symbolically it gave us permission to cry. Most of us did. Then he told us the clinical details. Reality therapy.

"Brenda went to bed last night around 8 p.m. She put a .357 magnum to her left temple and pulled the trigger," he said. "She died instantly."

"Had she been drinking?" asked someone.

"That would be speculation at this time," John answered. "I am sure they will check on it during the autopsy."

John went on. "As a point of information, I want to lay out an emotional road map for you. It can help reorient you."

Silence.

"First, there is the feeling no one else feels what you feel. There is a feeling of disbelief," he explained.

"I just can't believe it," said Jack.

"It isn't true," said Tim.

"It's got to be somebody's fault," said Rosie.

We repeated those phrases for weeks and months to come.

"What you need to understand is that all the emotions you feel are normal," said John. "This may be the first time you have felt them all at the same time."

"I hate her for what she did," said Michael. "If she was alive I think I'd kill her."

"I am so angry I'm sad." Nadine paused. "I'm glad she didn't suffer."

"I am afraid," said Julie.

"Expect those feelings to come and go," said John. "You know, it is a curious thing. My father died nine years ago. I found out with a phone call. Now every time the phone rings I think, 'Ah. It's Mom this time.' Part of my resolution over my loss is to recognize that my dad's death will be with me for my entire life."

More silence.

"When I heard it on the radio this morning," said Shirley, "it felt like the whole world was coming down on me. I can't remember driving to work. I drop everything I pick up." She knocked over my cup of coffee to emphasize her point.

"I know all of you are dealing with personal problems," said John. "This may make them seem worse."

"Mine seem smaller," said Pam.

"That is an interesting point," acknowledged John. He paused then he went on, "In tragedies like this we often relive a loss."

"I'm going to Brenda's funeral tomorrow," said Perry. "This is going to be tough." He blew his nose. "I attended her wedding last month. I just can't believe it. I keep seeing her sitting at her desk. Laughing. She was always laughing."

"I feel rotten," said someone.

"You need to understand, you are going to feel worse before you feel better," John told all of us.

"This sure is better than the last time," someone mumbled.

"What happened the last time?" asked John.

"Three years ago, a secretary overdosed on cocaine," Jack told John.

"No one talked about it," Nadine said. "We didn't know what to do."

John asked, "Anyone here reliving that now?"

Five hands went up.

Externally, Brenda's death seemed incongruent and impossible. John predicted, when the facts were known, it could be consistent with her life.

Three days before her suicide, she learned the baby she was expecting had Down's Syndrome—a mongoloid. Her previous two marriages had failed because she wasn't able to become pregnant.

Life had caved in on her at age 39. She chose not to look for the therapeutic support she had given to others. She forgot her own advice, "Never treat yourself."

People dealt with her suicide at the level they could deal with it. Some started rumors. Some blamed themselves. A whole bunch of people blamed me because I hadn't given her a big enough raise. I felt guilty, but at least I knew the facts. Confidentiality was her right. It may have been her demise.

Tim's proposal for expanded health promotion services was as disarming as Brenda's suicide, particularly after I had shut down *Healthy Habits* to avoid an imminent avalanche of debt. My decision to give health promotion one more chance was worth every penny.

New employee orientation now includes two health education workshops—CPR and PAINLESS, a program to prevent back pain. They introduce people to our organization's cultural belief: Good physical health means good fiscal health.

CPR is mandatory for everyone, every year, including me. Good thing for Roy. The blood pressure checks we do during each CPR class proved to be a good market research tactic as well.

We discovered 30 percent of our employees needed medical attention to control their blood pressure. We figured the rest of the city was probably in the same fix. We opened a *Health Hut* store at the regional shopping mall to screen shoppers for high blood pressure.

The store averages three admissions each week. If people have enough money to shop the mall, they tend to have insurance for vascular and heart surgery. We earned $189,000 in referral revenue from that tactic in the first six months of operation. Our back pain prevention class also has had a favorable financial impact. Worker compensation claims are down dramatically.

During PAINLESS class discussions we discovered our warehouse workers had no dollies or flatbeds to work with. In fact, most of our work stations were causing back injuries.

Our managers thought they were doing us a favor by delaying equipment purchases and living with the problems of poor design. What they didn't know was that each back injury cost us $50,000. Information changed their minds. Education improved their behavior. Good behavior pays for itself.

We ended up buying $12,000 worth of equipment. Our employees can now perform their jobs safely.

Our orientation classes have turned out well but our best idea has been a confidential counseling service, an Employee Assistance Program. So far we've salvaged four of our best managers and eight other good employees from alcohol and drug dependency problems. This is the same group of hospital employees who we didn't think had any problems.

If you don't take a temperature you won't find a fever.

Daily rounds—1:00 p.m.

Rounds are a good way to stay close to the customer. It's not the same experience I had as an orderly at Kettering Memorial Hospital in Dayton. No bed pans.

First stop was labor and delivery, the birthing place. There is a new batch of babies every day.

My father used to reminisce about his first delivery as an intern 50 years ago. The unwed mother's empty isolation etched an indelible memory for him. Mary was a 13-year-old girl who hadn't the slightest idea how she'd become pregnant. It was her second child. Not much has changed since 1933.

Teenage parents are as American as apple pie. I see a new one every day, usually two or three.

I hope we decide to eradicate the epidemic of unwanted pregnancy someday. Education is a vaccine that could solve the problem. Every child, aged 12 to 19, would have to present a signed statement from a doctor or nurse that would permit them to attend classes on the first day of each school year. The note would read:

_____ *knows how conception occurs, how sexually transmitted diseases can be prevented, and how pregnancies can be avoided.*
   *Signed*_____ MD/DO/RN

No note, no school.

"Good afternoon!" I said. "How's the birthing place today?"

"Fine except for the Hahn's baby," said Bertha, the head nurse. "We've got a full house. A couple of normal deliveries, a pair of C-sections, and one preemie we're going to send to the big city."

I can always tell when we have a preemie on the unit. Cigarette stink hangs in the air. Almost every preemie has a smoker for a mother. We are handsomely rewarded for ignoring the problem. The state pays us about $19,000 for every low weight baby we hospitalize. We collect $950 on a healthy delivery.

I looked around at all the happy faces. New parents. Grandparents. Great grandparents.

"Your staff has the best jobs in the hospital. Everyone smiles. Lots of action. Lots of satisfaction."

"Lots of malpractice."

"Did you get nailed this week, too?"

"My premium went from $59 to $502 a year. I almost fainted," said Bertha. "That's a 40-hour work week just to pay for coverage."

I thought about our new husband and wife obstetrical team. On top of a new office, new equipment, a new home, and four kids in school, they had to pay 85K for insurance. They have to deliver 365 babies a year to break even. 1988 was a leap year. They got to take a day off together. "Anybody else up here been hammered like that?" I asked.

"No," she said. "I'm shopping for a better rate. Maybe if I promise never to give my next door neighbors any advice ever again, they'll give me some slack."

My "buck-up, look-on-the-bright-side" pep talk was out of place. As I headed for the door, she quizzed me on my commitment to her prepared childbirth classes. "When are we going to get that replacement film for my classes?"

"It's in next year's capital budget."

"That's what you said last year."

"You're right. I apologize."

"I don't want an apology," Bertha argued. "Apologies are worthless if you don't mean them. We need that film. Don't you realize the contribution our prenatal education classes make in this community?"

"Yes, I do. I just don't think a $500 film is the answer. The plastic surgery trays we bought for breast implants knocked out a few frills. Your film was one of them," I said. "I really am sorry."

Bertha cocked her arm for a right cross.

"There isn't any incentive to educate parents," I backpedaled. "We could do a bang up job of prenatal education for about $900 per family if we had a mind to, but we need that money to pay your salary."

Intensive care unit—1:30 p.m.

A grim conversation blocked my entrance to ICU.

An attractive, slender woman about age 36 was crying. A neurologist held her left hand. Her diamond wedding band sparkled. She could have been a daughter, a sister, a mother, a grandmother, or an aunt. She could have been breaking down over a brother, a husband, an infant, an uncle, or a parent. Her love was wrapped around whoever was behind that door. Her tears said it all. Life was left in someone's lungs. Nothing was left between the ears.

"There's always a chance in cases like this," Dr. Rago said. "He may wake up. It's too soon to tell."

"It's been 110 days," she objected. "His brain waves are gone. His kidneys could help someone else."

"Mrs. O'Klessan, if we harvest his organs we would kill him."

"Kill him?" she despaired. "He has been dead since..."

"Excuse me please." I walked between them to enter the unit. Roy's ear-to-ear grin was the best thing I'd seen all day.

"How are you doing David?"

"Great," I said. "You're looking good. Give me five." Roy gave me five the way he slaps my 4-year-old son's hand. "I hear you're giving the nurses a hard time. I came down to straighten you out."

He looked much better than he did the night before. Pink cheeks.

"My chest hurts like the dickens."

"I bet it feels like you had a heart attack."

"It feels like somebody broke my ribs."

"I don't know how that could have happened," I said. "If you find the guy who did it, take my advice. Sue him."

We spoke about gardening, grandchildren, and the weather. It felt good to hold his hand. I watched the monitor bleeps—even, regular, and steady.

Roy whispered, "Look over there."

A birthday party. A cake and candles. They were singing happy birthday to Jimmy, a comatosed 33-year-old. Jimmy had bumped his head in a car accident. No broken bones. No bleeding. No seat belt.

Jimmy seized. His right hand waved.

"Oh look! Look!" said Jimmy's mother to Jimmy's dad. "He's never done that before."

I thought, "He used to do that all the time."

Roy gossiped, "His wife can't take much more of this. I heard her say he's been in here four months. What's the point?"

Jimmy's life did have meaning in an oddball sort of way. He was the hospital's best paying customer. The profit we earned from his insurance was paying us enough to cover the cirrhotic transient next to him and a fraction of the bill for the Hahn's baby. Jimmy's insurance company will raise its rates but we will keep our doors open.

ICU was full. Two gunshot wounds from Saturday night. Roy, Jimmy, and the Mexican. What a place.

I said, "Good-bye. See you tomorrow," and headed for the surgeon's lounge. As usual ICU nurses never have much time to talk. It's all business.

Surgeons' lounge—1:50 p.m.

This lounge is the 1980s' locker room version of an 1880s' men's club. Our female orthopods and gynecologists share the nurse's dressing rooms.

I poured myself a cup of stale coffee and felt how tired I was. If I was beat, how did Dr. Bob feel? He'd been here for 24 hours. His last surgery of the day, a triple bypass, had been bumped from 4:00 p.m. to 10:00 p.m. by an emergency double bypass. He finished the triple at 4:00 a.m. His routine work day begins at 7:00 a.m. sharp. He was glued to the tube on an ESPN Canadian log-rolling competition.

"You getting ready to head home?" I asked him.

"No." He shook his head.

I looked to a family doc for conversation.

"How's it going, Steve?"

"OK. Three vasectomies," he said.

"How come you didn't do them in your office?" I asked. "It's cheaper."

"Not if the insurance doesn't pay for it," he said. "For some reason, all three had coverage that required them to have their vas snipped in a hospital."

"Thanks," I said. "We appreciate the business."

"You're welcome."

Medical records—2:20 p.m.

"What's up?" I asked.

"Did you see the 5:00 p.m. news last night?" asked Janet.

"I wish. I had a meeting with the executive committee."

Janet, our medical records department head, had her malpractice insurance doubled to $160 a year. Now she is interested in every legal issue, large and small.

"Here's the scoop." Janet explained the situation. "An HMO enrollee needs a heart transplant. She doesn't think it's fair her insurance won't pay for it. She's paid all those premiums for all those years. She needs $475,000 and they won't help her. She took her case to Channel 12."

"What did they say?"

"Ten minutes of fluff. But their report may have created a problem for us."

"How so?"

"We admitted an employee's husband seven days ago. He needs Medicaid coverage. Apparently, she decided not to include him under our health plan."

"After he was admitted, they discovered he didn't fit any eligibility profile. No Medicaid assistance. No coverage. He's terminal."

"Let me guess." I thought of Jimmy. "We're eating a $12,878 bill. He's in pain. There isn't a nursing home within 200 square miles that will take him. She's deathly worried we will toss him out on the street."

"It's $13,457. He wants to die. His wife won't let him," Janet said. "She asked me if she should take her case to the papers. I thought you might want to know about it."

"Thanks a lot," I said. "Tell her we are on her side. We won't throw him out. We will do what's right."

"Glad to hear you say that again," said Janet. "It helps morale in the trenches."

"Glad to be of service," I said. "How old is he anyway?"

"Seventy-three. Usually guys with his DRG come in for one day, run up $7,950 worth of charges, and die. The ones who hang on forever drive us nutty."

"Anything else?"

"You bet. A discharge planning question," said Janet. "The guy we admitted last week who was found in a dumpster."

"The guy who disemboweled himself with a sardine can and then slit his throat?" I asked.

"That's the guy." She nodded her head. "He's being discharged today."

"So?"

"So isn't there anything we can do to protect him?"

"No one can protect a person from himself," I said. "I spoke with him three times. He told me it was an accident."

"Whoever did it is going to finish him off."

"Maybe. Maybe not. It is not a medical issue any more. Forget it."

"I can't."

"Neither can I, but we are both paid a lot of money to pretend we do."

Psychiatric care unit—3:05 p.m.

My last stop of the day was our children's behavioral medicine unit, psychiatric care for children. Larry, a paraprofessional counselor, looked worn and withdrawn. "What's up Larry?" I asked him. "Anger getting the best of the therapist in you?"

"You might say that," Larry said. "I want my innocence back."

"You can't have it."

"Damn," he said and blurted out his story. "I was giving little Kyle a bath. He was slapping his hand over his mouth like a 4-year-old Apache. Instead of a war whoop, he made a 'whop-whop-whop-whop-whop' sound.

"I asked him what that noise was. He said, 'humping noises.' I didn't think I heard him right. I asked him again. 'I said it's a humping noise.'

"I dried him off and brought him in here to play with these dolls." I followed him into a counseling room.

Larry handed me five anatomically correct Pumpkin Patch dolls. A white man. A black man. A Hispanic woman. A little white boy, and little Asian girl doll.

Larry explained therapy role play. "Kids don't get hung up on colors," he said. "They just name them daddy, mommy, me, and my sister. This time the man was 'my mommy's boyfriend.'

"So Kyle pulls off his 'mommy's' panties. He puts them on his head." Larry imitated Kyle. "He starts dancing around this room making the humping noise."

"I can't believe it."

"It's true. It makes me sick but it's true." said Larry. "Most of the kids in here tell these stories. I'm not even surprised anymore when I find out another one has VD.

"So then Kyle takes his 'mommy' and puts her mouth over his 'special purpose.' That's the word his mom told him to use. He takes his 'mommy's boyfriend' and puts a finger in his mommy's cookie and his thumb in her bum."

"You're exaggerating."

"Dolls don't lie."

"This sounds like a Penthouse letter."

"It's worse," said Larry. "The kid is only four. I ended his therapy session after his 'mommy' put a pencil up his bottom and told him to be a good boy."

"This is what you guys are dealing with?"

"Yeah, and that's not all of it." Larry was livid and his voice was loud. "The mommy's boyfriend is the same guy the DA plea-bargained with in that child pornography ring they busted last summer. He got off with three months."

"That can't be."

"It is," Larry insisted. "We wrote to everyone we could think of to keep him locked up. No one would help us."

"What are we going to do to help Kyle?" I asked.

"I called the Department of Social Services. We're going to try to get temporary, legal custody."

"That's almost impossible."

"I know. It's worth a try though. It will take us years to get a termination of parental rights judgment against her," he said. "It almost never happens. In a week or two Kyle will be back home."

"Is Kyle a Medicaid patient?"

"Yeah. And the last time we had a case like this Medicaid gave us a denial. No payment."

Home sweet home—4:45 p.m.

I canceled my 5 o'clock and 8 o'clock committee meetings. I was too tired to go on. A better way to run this business of health care has to be found.

6

WORLD CLASS HEALTH CARE

...my most fundamental objective is to urge a change in the perception and evaluation of familiar data.

Thomas S. Kuhn[1]

What was previously regarded as real, e.g., disease entities—may come to be looked upon as unreal, and what was previously taken to be unreal, e.g., curved space—may be admitted to reality. But when this happens the truth remains unaltered and new truth and old truth do not contradict.

C. I. Lewis[2]

It was as if the ground had been pulled out from under one, with no firm foundation to be seen anywhere, upon which one could have built.

Albert Einstein[3]

New Knowledge and the Scientific Revolution

Scientific revolution has occurred before. It will happen again. It is part of a natural progression, the human search for pure science.

Scientific disciplines progress through six stages. As summarized by Shewhart in his book, *Economic Control of Quality of Manufactured Product*,[4] they are:

1. Belief that the future cannot be predicted in terms of the past.
2. Belief that the future is preordained.
3. Inefficient use of past experience in the sense that experiences are not systematized into laws.
4. Control within limits.
5. Maximum control.
6. Knowledge of all laws of nature-exact science.

We think medicine's six stages can be described as:

1. Disease is completely unpredictable.
2. Disease is preordained.
3. Existing knowledge and experience is used inefficiently. Medical theory lacks sufficient integration.
4. Control is achieved within limits. Accurate predictions for health and illness become routine.
5. Maximum control is achieved. Health is built into the conception of life with good nutrition, a good lifestyle, and good stress management. Growth and maturation processes are made healthy through education, good health habits, health screenings, psychological support, and medical care.
6. Profound knowledge is achieved. Pure health science is mastered.

Medical science is in its infancy. It is poised for a leap from the third stage of insufficient integration to the fourth stage of controlled process. It will not jump of its own accord. Medical professionals whose productive careers grew from their commitment to tradition can be expected to resist any perceptual switch they think might derail their life's work.

A topsy-turvy perspective bewilders even the most brilliant individual. The revolutionary perception of medical science which will save millions of lives and billions of dollars mandates a transformation of the health care professions. It calls for a complete retooling of our health care industry.

The medical beliefs of our past and present are incapable of solving the health care puzzles of our future. Twentieth century medicine's noble history of achievements does not justify its continued use in the twenty-first century. That rationale must come from the answer to the $500 billion question, "Does it work?"

Today we must say, "Yes, but it benefits few at the expense of many." World Class Health Care works better. It benefits many at the expense of a few. Given a humane and wealthy society committed to caring for those few, World Class Health Care is the only choice our nation can make during the last decade of the twentieth century.

World Class Health Care's pragmatic approach has monetary value. The financial chaos of our nation's health care system juxtaposed to the promise of economical health care will persuade young minds to fly deep into the universe of health sciences. The rewards those students reap will spur others onto the learning curve. Learning will prompt practice and practice will develop great skill.

Their learning can result in profound knowledge only if students understand theory. Shewhart[5] emphasized this point when he wrote, "We cannot have facts without theory." Deming is less diplomatic: "People who have no theory don't know where they are going to."

The foundation of scientific revolution is new knowledge. Every physician, nurse educator, hospital administrator, or health care leader who adopts the quality approach must become familiar with the mathematics and philosophy of quality. Mastery of the quality discipline requires hard work and diligent study.

The quality philosophy demands a total commitment to scientific method. Statistical reasoning is a rigorous endeavor. The reward for dedication to scientific process and statistical reasoning is a completely unique, invigorating world view. The picture stirs a deep sense of order and interdependence. It intrigues and fascinates.

Einstein[3] was the first person to explain how an everyday person could get an abstract look at this view. Shewhart[4,5] gave us a tool which lets us touch the picture. Einstein's little book is a good place for any serious student of quality to begin. If our experience can serve as a guide, the reader should read all of these books[2-5] and should expect to read each book several times.

Quality health care, World Class Health Care, depends on the mathematics, philosophy, point of view, and ideas expressed in those books. We know of no shortcut. For the purposes of this book it is important to introduce the bones of Professor Lewis' outline of knowledge[2]. It is also necessary to review Shewhart's[5] notion about the three components of knowledge.

C. I. Lewis, Outline of a Theory of Knowledge

Professor Lewis summarized the first 273 pages of his book in two paragraphs[2].

> Quite commonly, the different types or phases of knowledge—presented objects, of a priori principles, of empirical generalizations—are all lumped together, and either what is true of one type only is applied to all, where in some other

fashion an omnibus explanation is attempted which will include them all under one formula. No theory devised by such procedure can ever be more than partially successful.

The following need to be distinguished: (1) the immediate awareness of the given, such as might be supposed to be reported in statements like, "This looks round," "This feels hard," "This tastes sweet"; (2) knowledge of presented objects, such as expressed by, "This is *hard*," "This is a sweet apple," "This penney is round"; (3) the a priori elaboration of wholely abstract concepts, like the formulations of pure mathematics, apart from any question of possible applications; (4) the categorical knowledge of interpretive principles and criteria of reality, which is that form of a priori knowledge which arises when concepts have a fixed denotation and are applied to the given; (5) empirical generalizations, which are universal but not a priori.

When a disease process (an object in Lewis and Shewhart's language) "presents itself" practitioners commonly lump together the old knowledge of the current medical model. Doctors assume the genesis is organic. A variety of empirical generalizations are automatically made from this presumption. Those generalizations inevitably result in medical intervention, surgical intervention, or both. The artistic blend of these decisions is largely based upon the patient's ability to pay for services, clinical memory, and litigation paranoia.

This approach to diagnosis and treatment is seldom more than partially successful. It often results in perpetual treatment. Hospitals serve to remind us of this fact.

The World Class Health Care practitioner takes a more scientific approach. Each phase of knowledge is addressed independently.

1. When a disease process presents itself the practitioner becomes aware of it.

    This person looks ill.

2. The illness is operationally defined using good data collection technique.

    This person is injured. The injury has lifestyle, mental, and physical origins. Specifically, there is evidence of alcohol and tobacco use. There is depression. There is a broken leg.

3. The World Class Health Care giver has knowledge of variation, formal distribution theory, and probability theory.

4. Control charts are used to determine the state of statistical control. Original data are graphed in sequence so patterns and groupings of data become visible. Probabilities are calculated.

5. Empirical generalizations based on a familiarity with the patient's disease process and its state of statistical control can be made as follows:

> Alcohol abuse caused the broken leg. We must first fix the leg. We must then work to minimize alcohol abuse so further trauma is avoided. We must also relieve the depression and eliminate the use of tobacco so a return to the hospital can be avoided.

W. A. Shewhart, Three Components of Knowledge[5]

Shewhart began his outline of the three components of knowledge by quoting C. I. Lewis.[2]

> I shall assume that knowledge begins and ends in experimental data but that it does not end in the data in which it begins.

Shewhart[4,5] felt that:

> From this viewpoint, there are three important components of knowledge: (a) the data of experience in which the process of knowing *begins*, (b) the prediction P in terms of data that one would expect to get if he were to perform certain experiments in the *future*, and (c) the degree of belief pb in the prediction P based on the original data or some summary thereof as evidence E... knowledge begins in the original data and ends in the data predicted, these future data constituting the operationally verifiable meaning of the original data.

Shewhart's[4,5] point of view met Lewis' criteria for logic, "A good logic must be circular." Circular logic is apparent in the Shewhart-Deming cycle. It also surfaces in his illustration of the three interlocking components of knowledge (Figure 6.1).

Shewhart wrote, "to every prediction there corresponds a certain degree of rational belief." He was aware that humans have no quantitative way of measuring belief but "the results of an experiment should be presented in a way to contribute most readily to the development of the knowing "process."[5] To Shewhart an economic standard of quality is not a written finality but is a dynamic process. "It is not merely the imprisonment of the past in the form of a specification (Step I) but rather the unfolding of the future as revealed in the process of production (Step II) and inspection (Step III) and made available in the running quality report."[5]

Shewhart's circular logic and statistical theory found its first home in manufacturing. It will find a second home in health care because the economic standard of health care quality is also a dynamic process. It is a process which should continue until there is evidence found in Step III, the judgment of quality (Figure 3.1), which indicates that the desired specification, resilient good health, has been achieved. The health care

```
Original data as ─────────────── Prediction P
  Evidence E  \                    /
               \                  /
                \                /
                 \              /
                  Degree of belief pb
                  in Prediction P
                  based on evidence E
```

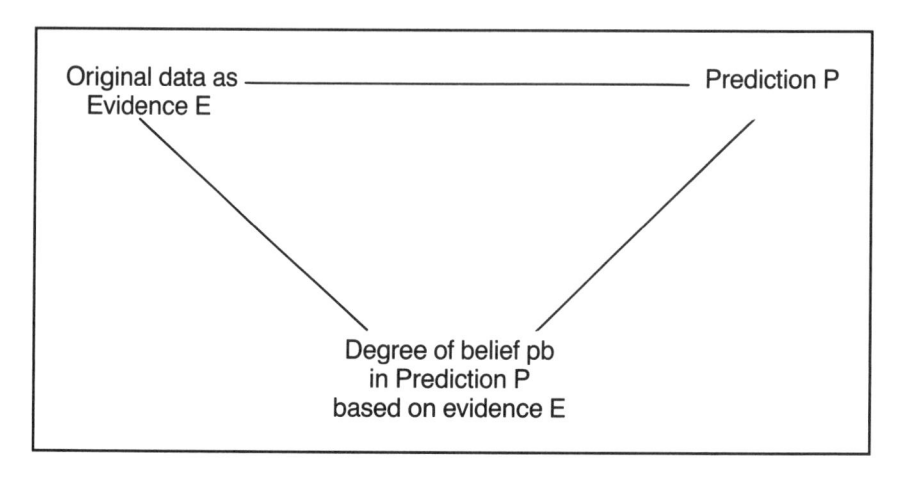

Figure 6.1 Shewhart's three interlocking components of knowledge. *Used with permission of the American Society for Quality Control. Walter Shewhart,* Statistical Method from the Viewpoint of Quality Control, *page 86.*

industry must have more to do with the "knowing process" of health. Health care must moderate its obsession with the content of a particular "medical" problem viewed in isolation from the process which produced the problem.

Shewhart saw the importance of minimizing the economic losses which result from tampering. That is, taking action on a process without knowledge of its state of statistical control. Health care givers also need to understand this principle of quality economics. Tampering, treating a process output (disease or trauma) as if it were a special cause rather than a common cause or vice versa, causes chaos. Accurate prediction becomes impossible. The results are huge losses to society. Tampering has led us into health care chaos.

Comment

Medical science in the late twentieth century is a single-stringed instrument with a capacity for sounding a five-note scale. World Class Health Care promises a six-string guitar—acoustic, electric, and engineered to produce every sound and tonal quality imaginable. Those of us who have heard it know the music is irresistible.

The market demand for such an instrument, once heard, boggles the mind. When the market realizes that World Class Health Care can be profitably priced well below the existing product, lines will stretch around the globe.

The world can then experience vastly improved levels of health care measured by substantial reductions in the incidence of illness. Recoveries will be speedy. The costs of quality health care will plummet.

Reduced costs will free up the investment money health science needs for education, prevention, the development of superior diagnostic protocols, and efficient treatment plans. This is a brighter future than the grim one guaranteed by our present health care model: (1) exclusion from service for all but the well-insured and well-to-do, (2) erratic and irrational rationing of treatment, and (3) extraordinary technology expenditures made for ever-diminishing returns.

In 1990 education, mental health services, and prevention are sacrificed to "lower" health care costs. Ironically, these are the very elements of health science which can lead us into a healthier future. They can give our health care industry the capacity for quality.

The courage and wisdom it takes to fund the development of these essential services comes with a cursory understanding of World Class Health Care. World Class Health Care is in the patient's best interest. It is also in the health care purchaser's best interest.

Medical tradition maintains an almost invincible seller's market. World Class Health Care turns health care into a buyer's market. The patient is the customer who will be king. When the patients and buyers decide to exert their influence, affordable prices become an expected health care characteristic. Even the poorest citizens in our nation's rural and urban communities will be able to access adequate and appropriate care.

The KAIZEN Principle—
Gradual, Incremental, Continuous Improvement

The product design changes required to shift our health care industry's focus from economic needs to patient care needs demand innovative thinking. People in search of stability resent innovation and change. People charged with the responsibility of preserving jobs battle against it unless they understand the principles of KAIZEN.

The Japanese word KAIZEN[7] summarizes the international management philosophy of continuous, incremental quality improvements (Figure 6.2). It is an excellent word to use for describing an awareness and respect for the forces of process.

KAIZEN faith generates the quiet, supreme confidence which comes from knowing quality lives in the heart of process. KAIZEN means knowing in your bones that quality pays. Its tangible dividends include job security, the creation of new jobs, increased profits, ever-increasing productivity, delighted customers, and long-term survival.

KAIZEN faith creates missionary zeal. KAIZEN is the catalyst for improved attitudes and behaviors. These in turn facilitate constant change for the better, constant improvement of quality. KAIZEN-conscious service

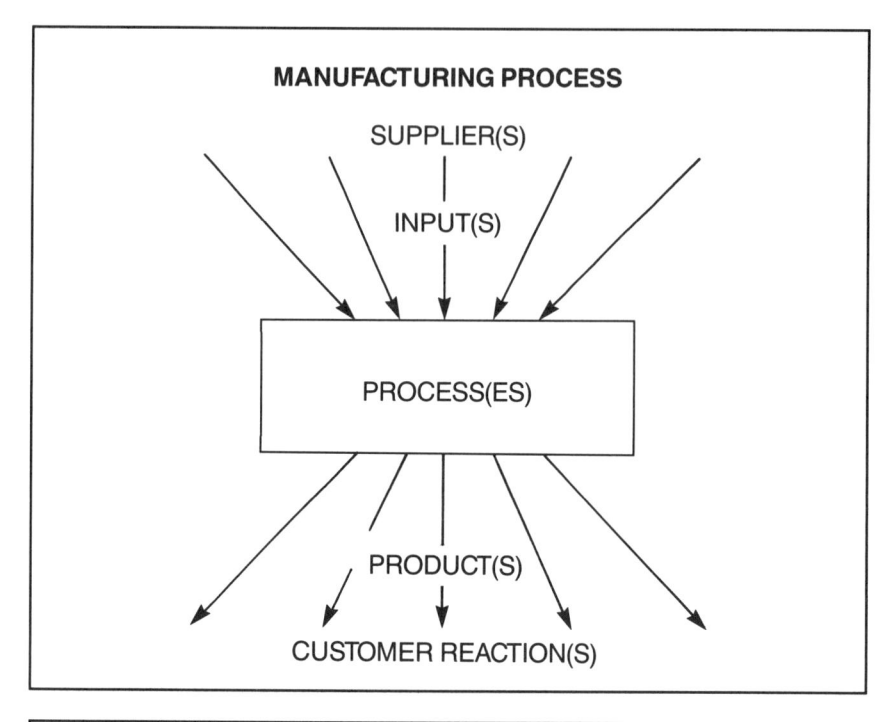

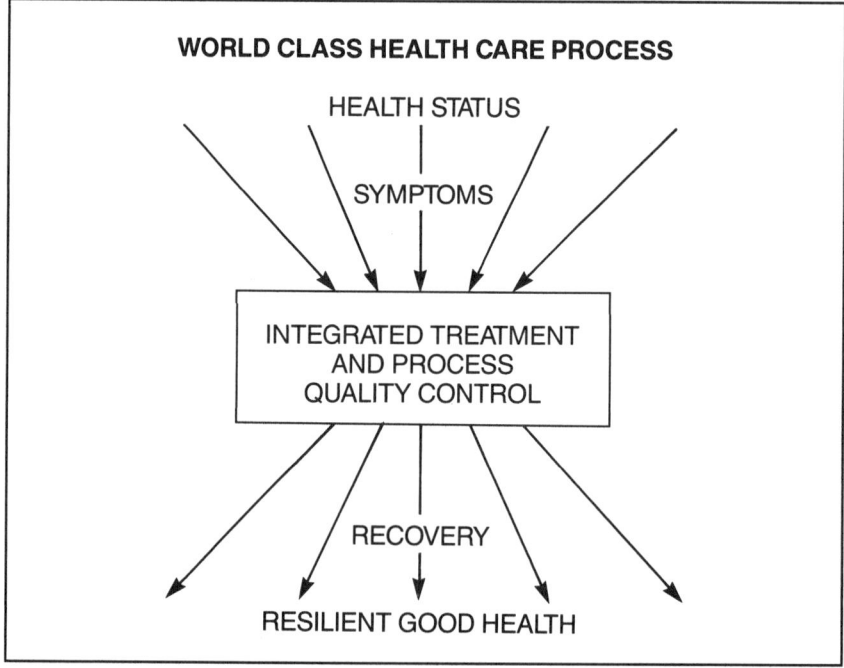

Figure 6.2 Principles of KAIZEN as applied in manufacturing and World Class Health Class. *Adapted with permission of McGraw-Hill from* Juran's Quality Control Handbook, Fourth Edition, *page 6.20.*

workers become proud enough to brag about and buy the services they deliver.

The stress of enormous expense is making the unconscious battle to preserve the past a troubling one for care givers. It tortures health care managers who fail to grasp the significance of KAIZEN and the continuous quality improvement process. The medical industry's foundation was not built to withstand this kind of political and economic force.

Rapid change is possible and durable but no elected government can be expected to initiate it. Hospitals which are stuggling to survive can be asked to use World Class Health Care, but hospitals take their marching orders from our government. A health care system based upon education, prevention, accurate diagnosis, integrated treatment, and statistical process control will cause our elected officials and our medical industrial complex pain. This pain can best be borne by going slowly but surely in the direction of good health.

Managing the Change to Quality Health Care

Any person who presents a medical problem now, particularly one requiring hospitalization, is in trouble. These patients have a right to expect an accurate and complete diagnosis. They have a right to expect cost-effective treatment. Today's patient care falls woefully short on both counts because the a priori assumption of our medical model—the genesis of disease is organic—clouds the patient's and the care giver's ability to think freely. It blurs their ability to reason. It flaws data collection methodology.

Mental health and lifestyle data are routinely omitted from the diagnostics of Medical Tradition. Psychotherapy and education are considered to be expensive, superfluous treatment. But an efficient, cost-effective health sciences process must include medical science, behavioral science, education, and statistical disciplines.

Prior to the 1980s' prospective payment system of Diagnostic Related Groups (DRGs), physicians worked as independent patient managers. Their extraordinary set of problem-solving skills was unfettered by fiscal restraint. Good medicine was measured by adherence to the well-defined rules of physical assessment, prescribed medical or surgical treatments, and evaluation. The medical doctor made all treatment decisions.

To its detriment, this "captain of the ship" doctrine became extremely profitable. Those profits fueled an inflation rate for medical services far exceeding our nation's norm. Even worse, they weakened medicine's commitment to the prevention of medical problems. For some, compassion and concern over the plight of the human condition began at the point of payment, not before. This patient path is diagrammed in Figure 6.3.

The cost of this logic invited the participation of additional patient managers who would limit expenditures. The DRG prospective payment system "capped" medical resource allocations. It linked a review of rationed resources (utilization review) directly to payment for services. If resources

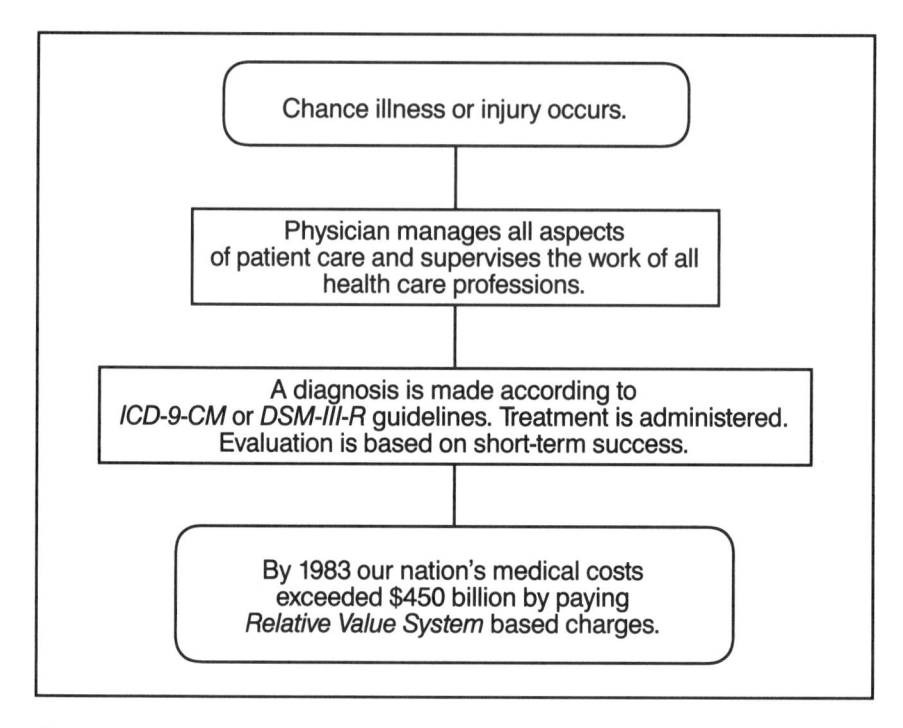

```
┌─────────────────────────────────────────────────────┐
│         ╭─────────────────────────────╮             │
│         │  Chance illness or injury    │            │
│         │         occurs.              │            │
│         ╰─────────────────────────────╯             │
│                      │                              │
│         ┌─────────────────────────────┐             │
│         │  Physician manages all aspects │          │
│         │ of patient care and supervises│          │
│         │   the work of all health     │           │
│         │     care professions.        │           │
│         └─────────────────────────────┘             │
│                      │                              │
│    ┌──────────────────────────────────────┐         │
│    │    A diagnosis is made according to   │        │
│    │ ICD-9-CM or DSM-III-R guidelines.    │         │
│    │    Treatment is administered.         │        │
│    │ Evaluation is based on short-term     │        │
│    │           success.                    │        │
│    └──────────────────────────────────────┘         │
│                      │                              │
│         ╭─────────────────────────────╮             │
│         │   By 1983 our nation's medical│           │
│         │   costs exceeded $450 billion │           │
│         │        by paying              │           │
│         │ Relative Value System based   │           │
│         │          charges.             │           │
│         ╰─────────────────────────────╯             │
└─────────────────────────────────────────────────────┘
```

Figure 6.3 Outline of patient path of medical tradition before 1980s diagnostic related groups' prospective payment system.

were misused, payment was withheld. Second opinions became mandatory for certain elective procedures.

The government's prospective DRG payment schedule forced shorter hospital stays. Case mix management which combined and correlated medical record data on an individual basis with the patient's bill, shamed providers by relating costs to price. Utilization review passed judgment on the appropriateness of health services. Second opinions made doctors think twice.

Taken together these tactics restricted access to care. They failed to contain our nation's growing health care bill. They failed to improve the quality of care. Rising costs and recurrent illness are in full bloom.

The patient path, revised by cost containment and mass inspection, diagrammed in Figure 6.4, bears a striking resemblance to its predecessor.

The fly in the 1980s' cost-containment ointment is the same one that has buzzed around our heads since publication of *International Classification of Diseases*[9] and *The Diagnostic and Statistical Manual*.[10] The *Relative Value System (RVS)* institutionalized four faulty deductions based on a theoretical a priori assumption: there is an organic genesis for disease.

```
┌─────────────────────────────────────────────────────────┐
│              ╭─────────────────────────╮                │
│              │  Chance illness or injury.│               │
│              ╰─────────────────────────╯                │
│                          │                              │
│  ┌───────────────────────────────────────────────────┐  │
│  │ Physicians share patient management and supervision│ │
│  │  responsibilities. Patient managers comply with    │ │
│  │ prospective payment restrictions, utilization review,│
│  │         and second opinion requirements            │  │
│  └───────────────────────────────────────────────────┘  │
│                          │                              │
│    ┌─────────────────────────────────────────────┐      │
│    │ A diagnosis is made according to ICD-9-CM or DSM-III-R │
│    │      guidelines. Treatment is administered.   │     │
│    │     Evaluation is based on short-term success.│     │
│    └─────────────────────────────────────────────┘      │
│                          │                              │
│    ╭─────────────────────────────────────────────╮      │
│    │     By 1988 our nation's health care expenditures │ │
│    │   exceed $500 billion by paying Relative Value System│
│    │                 based charges.              │      │
│    ╰─────────────────────────────────────────────╯      │
└─────────────────────────────────────────────────────────┘
```

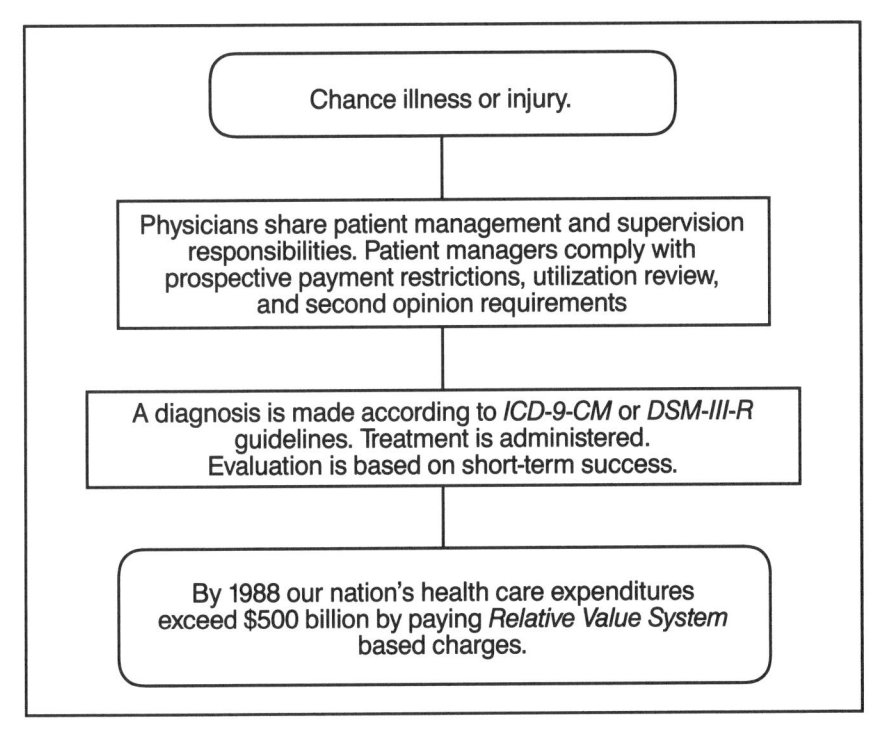

Figure 6.4 Patient path of medical tradition revised by cost containment and mass inspection resembles its predecessor

- The medical doctor is trained to collect and analyze all data required for an accurate diagnosis.
- The medical model for diagnosis ought to serve as the sole rationale for reimbursement.
- Physical science, medical and surgical technique ought to command a higher monetary value than behavioral science, education, and prevention.
- Patient behavior ought to be ignored or excused. Patients ought not to be expected to change the thinking or health habits which cause and maintain medical problems.

Health care providers are praised and rewarded for close adherence to the prevailing philosophy. Any etiology which cannot be measured by the gold standards of auscultation, palpation, visual assessment, chemistry, or diagnostic imaging doesn't count.

If those of us in health care have learned anything, we have learned diagnostic labels are misleading symptom descriptions. Thought, attitude, emotion and behavior, none of which can be adequately measured by the physical sciences, cause 50 percent or more of all hospitalizations. These hospital admissions must be classified as bad outcomes; they are evidence of poor quality care. These hospitalizations must be considered as defects to be minimized and eliminated from the health care process.

The Surgeon General's report[11] and the Carter Center Study[12] are but two bits of cogent evidence which support this fact. The personal losses each of us has experienced within our own families are far more persuasive.

Every citizen in the United States knows someone who has been crippled by a chosen lifestyle, someone who has died a tobacco, alcohol, or drug-related death. We must remember what we know about ourselves.

The presentation of an illness or injury is generally not a bit of bad luck. Most variations in health are caused. Medical or surgical problems, particularly ones which require a hospitalization, are often teachable moments in a highly predictable pattern of misbehavior and psychological distress. The teachable moment of hospitalization can and should be used to the patient's and the health care purchaser's advantage. It can and should result in the long-term resolution of three problems.

1. The immediate medical/surgical problem must be treated effectively enough to prevent a relapse.
2. A patient's psychological and emotional health must be balanced.
3. Patient thoughts and behaviors must be labeled and changed so a return to the hospital is avoided.

None of these can be achieved as long as we use the most expensive and least intrusive treatment. The most expensive treatment is preferred because it produces profit. The least intrusive treatment is preferred by patients because nobody wants their thinking or their lifestyle to be disturbed.

Both choices are understandable but rising costs are pricing medical services out of everyone's reach. Self-destructive thinking and lifestyles usually need to be disrupted to bring about lasting recoveries. Mental and emotional health problems need to be treated if we are to solve medical problems in a cost-effective manner.

The World Class Health Care Process

The flow diagram in Figure 6.5 must be legislated into action. It must serve as a precondition of payment for services. It can deliver higher quality, less expensive care. When used as the standard treatment protocol, the World Class Health Care process can save millions of lives and billions of dollars.

This blueprint can do more than reduce our nation's acute care health costs. It can solve our nation's cost/access/quality puzzle. It can improve the quality of health care services far beyond accepted industry standards.

The new treatment process cannot replace the old process unless it

WORLD CLASS HEALTH CARE

Predictable illness occurs. Hospitalization required.

Physical Science Assessment by Medical Doctor

Behavioral Science Assessment by Psychologist

Lifestyle Assessment by Nurse Educator

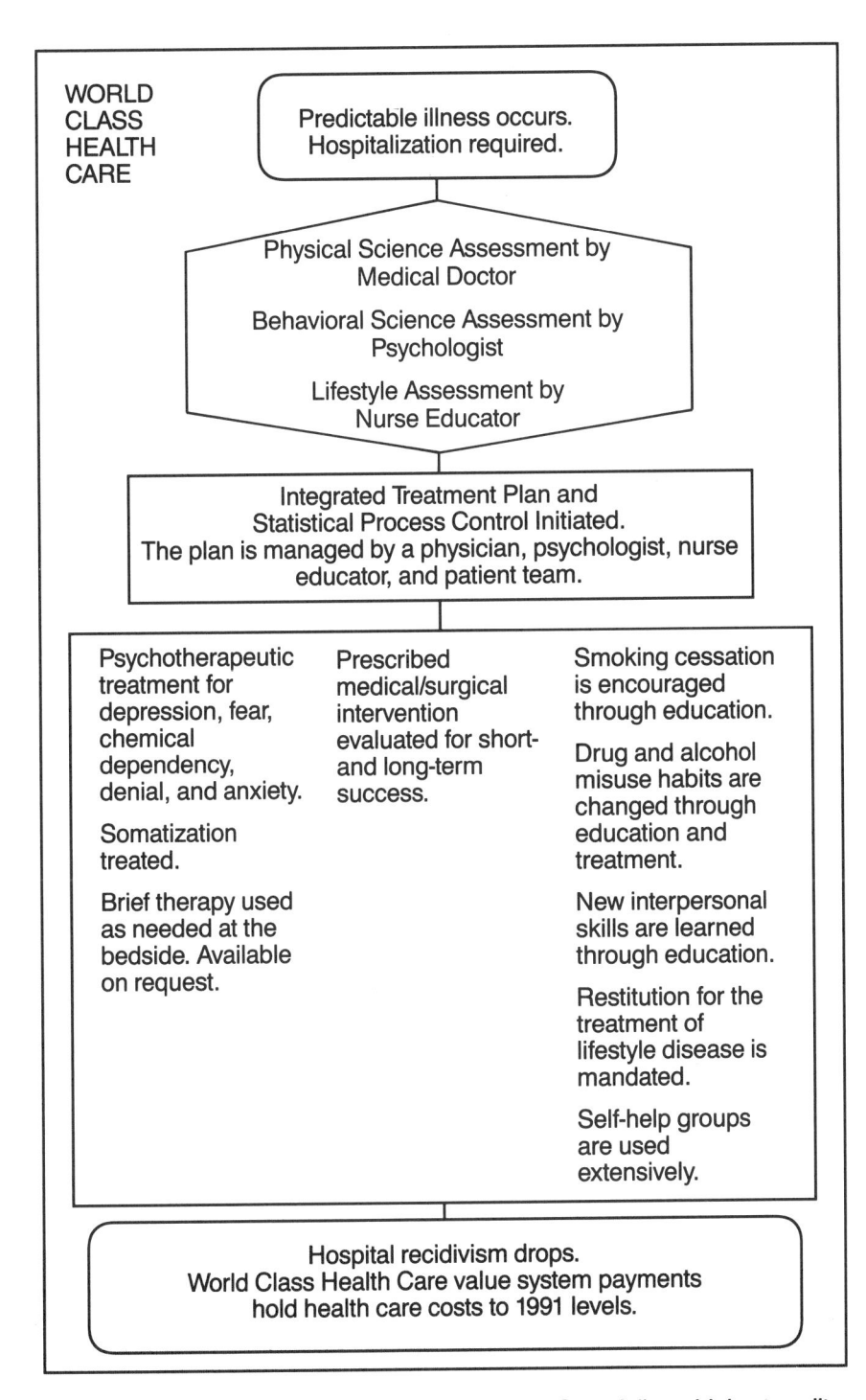

Integrated Treatment Plan and Statistical Process Control Initiated. The plan is managed by a physician, psychologist, nurse educator, and patient team.

Psychotherapeutic treatment for depression, fear, chemical dependency, denial, and anxiety.

Somatization treated.

Brief therapy used as needed at the bedside. Available on request.

Prescribed medical/surgical intervention evaluated for short- and long-term success.

Smoking cessation is encouraged through education.

Drug and alcohol misuse habits are changed through education and treatment.

New interpersonal skills are learned through education.

Restitution for the treatment of lifestyle disease is mandated.

Self-help groups are used extensively.

Hospital recidivism drops. World Class Health Care value system payments hold health care costs to 1991 levels.

Figure 6.5 Patient path using World Class Health Care delivers highest quality, lowest total cost care.

promises new value and attractive rewards. The idea market works the same as any other place of exchange: customers buy benefit. World Class Health Care can deliver on its promises. It can raise the quality of care, lower the total costs of care, and improve access to health care services. Each of the five segments in our proposed treatment flow diagram carries quality and value-added service to the patient.

Benefit: Hope Replaces Fear (Figure 6.6)

```
┌─────────────────────────────────┬─────────────────────────────────┐
│       FROM FIGURE 6.4           │       FROM FIGURE 6.5           │
│       Medical Tradition         │     World Class Health Care     │
│                                 │                                 │
│   Chance illness or injury.     │   Predictable illness occurs.   │
│                                 │   Hospitalization required.     │
└─────────────────────────────────┴─────────────────────────────────┘
```

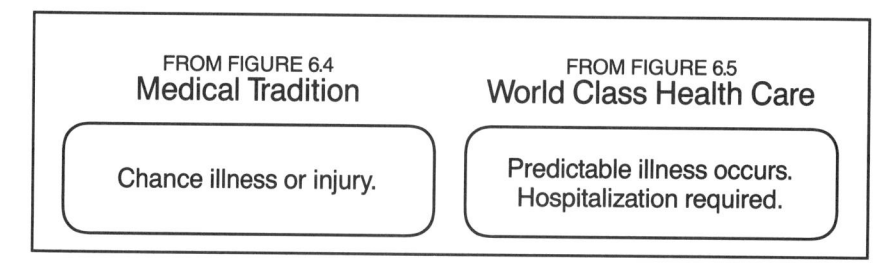

Figure 6.6 World Class Health Care replaces fear with hope.

Medical Tradition assumes illness is unpredictable. Uncertainty frightens us. The absence of control terrifies us. Chance illness is a premise which fosters fear.

World Class Health Care givers know that many hospitalizations are self-selective. They know the Carter Center Study[12] results are correct; many hospitalizations can be prevented.

The quality approach of World Class Health Care has the power to turn prevention into a scientific, common sense way of life. The knowledge which grows from the quality philosophy nourishes a sense of control, empowerment, and personal responsibility.

World Class Health Care taps an infinite resource, continuous knowledge. Knowledge can reduce the demand for technology-intensive services. Knowledge can help us avoid the rationing of finite resources.

Roy's heart attack, Mrs. Jameson's surgery, Mr. Pitstick's CT scan, Mr. Martin's emergency room visit, and tens of thousands of other hospital admissions are predictable events. We can break this tragic routine by breaking the conceptual boundaries which bind us to waste and inefficiency.

Benefit: Team Judgment Replaces Individual Opinion (Figure 6.7)

Medical Tradition presumes the unassailable superiority of independent physician judgment while it assumes the presence of an uneducated public.

World Class Health Care acknowledges the professional peer relationship which exists between medicine, behavioral science, and education. It applies the knowledge of a well-informed population.

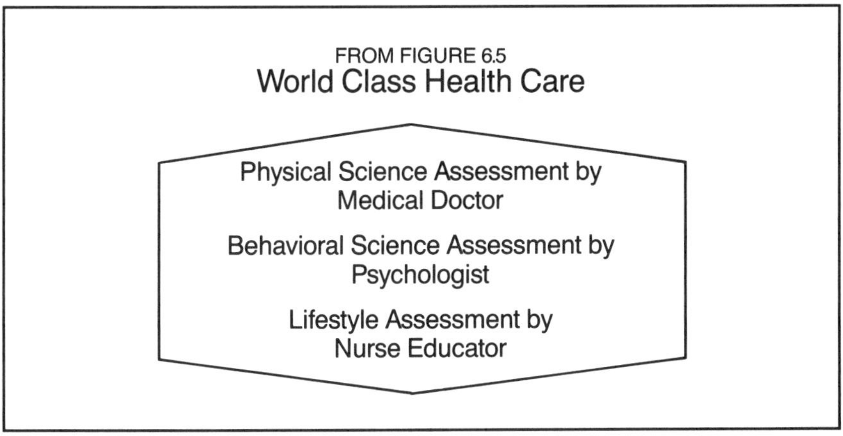

```
┌─────────────────────────────────────────────────┐
│              FROM FIGURE 6.5                    │
│           World Class Health Care               │
│                     ___                         │
│          ┌─────────────────────────┐            │
│          │ Physical Science Assessment by │     │
│          │      Medical Doctor            │     │
│          │                                │     │
│          │ Behavioral Science Assessment by│    │
│          │       Psychologist              │    │
│          │                                 │    │
│          │ Lifestyle Assessment by         │    │
│          │    Nurse Educator               │    │
│          └─────────────────────────┘            │
└─────────────────────────────────────────────────┘
```

Figure 6.7 World Class Health Care acknowledges the professional peer relationship between medicine, behavioral science, and education.

Any plan, including a health care treatment plan, requires prediction. Any plan which involves people requires precise operational definitions and clear communication. Data framed by statistical process control provides a common language and a sound basis for prediction.

Shifting the charter for diagnosis and assessment from the individual medical practitioner to a multidisciplinary treatment team will be strenuous work. The challenge conquered ratifies a health care Magna Carta.

Patients who enter the World Class Health Care system will enjoy unprecedented guarantees and opportunities for good health which cannot exist in the belief system of medical traditions.

Benefit: Balance Replaces Bias (Figures 6.8 and 6.9)

Medical Tradition diagnostic protocols rely on intuitive, arbitrary, narrow, and generally incomplete data gathering. Wide variations in diagnosis and treatment result from this process. (Figure 6.8).

World Class Health Care insists on scientific process discipline, unbiased data collection, and patient participation. It requires the use of statistical process control to integrate medicine, behavioral science, and education. Well structured, standardized processes reduce variations, thereby improving quality. (Figure 6.9).

Benefit: Problem Resolution Replaces the Quick Fix (Figures 6.10 and 6.11)

Medical Tradition spares neither time nor expense to break out the technology and "solve" a problem pronto. A vast industry has been built on the bedrock of impulsive action (Figure 6.10).

> **FROM FIGURE 6.4**
> **Medical Tradition**
>
> > Physicians share patient management and supervision responsibilities. Patient managers comply with prospective payment restrictions, utilization review, and second opinion requirements.

Figure 6.8 Traditional diagnostic protocols rely on intuitive, narrow, and incomplete data gathering. Wide variations in treatment result.

> **FROM FIGURE 6.5**
> **World Class Health Care**
>
> > Integrated Treatment Plan and Statistical Process Control Initiated.
> > The plan is managed by a physician, psychologist, nurse educator, and patient team.

Figure 6.9 World Class Health Care insists on scientific process discipline, unbiased data collection, and patient participation. Standardized processes reduce variation, thereby improving quality.

> **FROM FIGURE 6.4**
> **Medical Tradition**
>
> > A diagnosis is made according to *ICD-9-CM* or *DSM-III-R* guidelines. Treatment is administered.
> > Evaluation is based on short-term success.

Figure 6.10 Medical tradition spares neither time nor expense to "solve" a problem.

World Class Health Care uses deliberate thought and coordinated action. It values the benefits of short-term problem solutions but not at the expense of the desired outcome, resilient good health. Education is fundamental to every treatment as is therapy for the psychological distress which causes, accompanies, and results from illness (Figure 6.11).

FROM FIGURE 6.5
World Class Health Care

Psychotherapeutic treatment for depression, fear, chemical dependency, denial, and anxiety.

Somatization treated.

Brief therapy used as needed at the bedside. Available on request.

Prescribed medical/surgical intervention evaluated for short- and long-term success.

Smoking cessation is encouraged through education.

Drug and alcohol misuse habits are changed through education and treatment.

New interpersonal skills are learned through education.

Restitution for the treatment of lifestyle disease is mandated.

Self-help groups are used extensively.

Figure 6.11 World Class Health Care uses deliberate thought and coordinated action.

The omission of either behavioral science, education, or the statistical tools of process quality control is an unconscionable compromise World Class Health Care is unwilling to make. Patients and care givers alike will benefit from their collegial relationship and shared responsibility for outcome. Integrity, trust, cooperation, and mutual respect will put the monster of malpractice to death.

Benefit: Cost-Effective Treatment Replaces Perpetual Treatment

The economic lifeblood of Medical Tradition is the *Relative Value System* (*RVS*) and its newborn cousin the *Resource-Based Relative Value Scale*

(*RBRVS*). Both payment systems channel a Mississippi-sized river of revenue to technology-intensive (i.e., expensive) diagnostic, medical, and surgical interventions. Their perverse incentives often reward inadequate and inappropriate treatment. They drive routine health care management decisions; hospitalize and use technology whenever possible (Figure 6.12).

FROM FIGURE 6.4
Medical Tradition

In 1988 our nation's health care expenditures exceed $500 billion by paying *Relative Value System* based charges.

Figure 6.12 The Relative Value System rewards inadequate and sometimes inappropriate treatment.

World Class Health Care places the highest value on thinking. A World Class Health Care system mandates equal pay for equal work. The skill, thinking, and stress associated with the delivery of the care required to keep people well equals the skill, thinking, and stress of repairing the damage done by lifestyle and disease.

Paying a care giver for the time spent in thought about a patient's health makes sense. Paying that same care giver four times the amount of money, for the same amount of time, when he or she thinks inside a hospital is nonsense. It invites abuse.

The disparity in pay scales between the health professions is a barrier which must be gradually dismantled. Educator, behavioral scientist, and physician cognitive skills are of equal value to the patient. The work to be done is primarily statistical thinking, prevention, education, and mental and physical health maintenance (Figure 6.13).

FROM FIGURE 6.5
World Class Health Care

Hospital recidivism drops.
World Class Health Care value system payments hold health care costs to 1991 levels.

Figure 6.13 With World Class Health Care education, behavioral scientist, and physician cognitive skills are of equal value to the patient.

The incomes to be earned in the process of delivering health care will be made mostly before an admission to the hospital occurs.

When a good living can be made from producing good health, the aggressive treatment of terminal illnesses will become less fashionable. Hospitals can play a critically important leadership role during the transition phase of the next 20 years. Those institutions which can demonstrate character and intergrity will prosper while they redefine their missions. Two case study examples compare the use of World Class Health Care to Medical Tradition in Appendix B.

Hospitalization As a Teachable Moment

Every person in our country eventually uses one or more hospital services during his or her lifetime. A hospital is the safest place for childbirth, corrective surgeries, and the treatment of serious psychiatric problems. Some hospitalizations for accidents, infections, and age are unavoidable. But the Surgeon General's report[11] and Carter Center Study[12] remind us that many hospital admissions are related to lifestyle. They can and should be prevented.

Hospitalizations are teachable moments. They deserve the most effective treatment available. The three laws of learning defined by the pioneer psychologist Edward L. Thorndike[13] (1874–1949) can put more power into the practice of medicine.

- The law of readiness is self-evident. People must be ready to learn before learning occurs. They must be motivated.
- The law of effect predicts people will repeat behaviors which are satisfying. Rewards are important to learning.
- The law of frequency is one of the precious few truths in life; people must practice skills in order to master them.

People pay attention when they think they are in danger of dying. Three fail-safe motivators always grab a person's attention and get a person ready to learn: hope, fear, and money. These three are everywhere in a hospital.

A hospitalization is a frightening confrontation with one's past and present. Although fear is only a short-term motivator, it exposes the survival instinct and presents care givers with a singular opportunity to harness the power of hope.

Money can effect quick, temporary behavior changes. Money in the form of technology, education, behavioral science, shared risk and responsibility can change long-term, lifestyle behavior. Money can drive the care giver's desire to teach and the patient's desire to be well as surely as it drives their desires to treat and be treated. Clearly defined exclusions and limitations to subsidized treatment for chronic lifestyle and terminal-end stage diseases will strengthen the effect. Financial incentives for compliance with treatment plans and penalties for noncompliance can instill essential teamwork between patients and care givers. When we choose to reward health instead of illness, we will find more than enough money in our health care system to motivate everyone.

Each piece of the World Class Health Care flow diagram builds quality into the health care process. Putting the pieces together is a sensible, albeit formidable, thing to do. The contributions medical and surgical treatment can make to the treatment team are well documented and accepted.

The contributions behavioral science, education, and statistical process control can make are well documented. They are rejected or met with indifference only because they lie slightly beyond the insular boundaries of obsolete medical beliefs. The treatment team can move the boundaries by using World Class Health Care for every hospitalization.

Integrated Treatment

Integrated treatment calls for teamwork. The integrated treatment team (physician, psychologist, nurse educator, and patient) has the potential for four-dimensional vision and analysis. A more thoughtful treatment plan can be developed when the number of diagnosticians increases from one to four.

Every team needs a leader. The rigor of the medical doctor's education will safeguard the physician's status as team captain but physician responsibilities shall change dramatically. Psychologists and nursing trained health educators must be peers with equal decision-making authority. The patient is the fourth and all-important treatment team member.

Equally shared responsibility all but eliminates the possibility of a malpractice lawsuit. Every outcome hinges on the level of physical and mental health a patient brings to the treatment process. Certainly few patients will decide to sue themselves for misjudgment or misbehavior.

The treatment team has three equally important goals: (1) restore physical health, (2) restore psychological health, and (3) establish habits to maintain health. The team will be required to work within a predetermined budget which is known to all team members. Patients who comply with treatment plan recommendations will be charged substantially less than patients who refuse to participate in their recovery. Patients who follow team decisions will be able to access technology intensive resources. Patients who choose not to follow treatment guidelines will lose their right to access those resources. Everyone on the team will be obligated to use statistical methods from the viewpoint of quality control.

The Shewhart-Deming cycle[4-6] is an ideal process model for the team to use during the course of treatment (Figure 6.14). The plan must be based on fact. Every hospitalization must include a complete physical, psychological, and lifestyle behavior assessment. Ideally, every visit to a doctor's office should include the same approach to data collection.

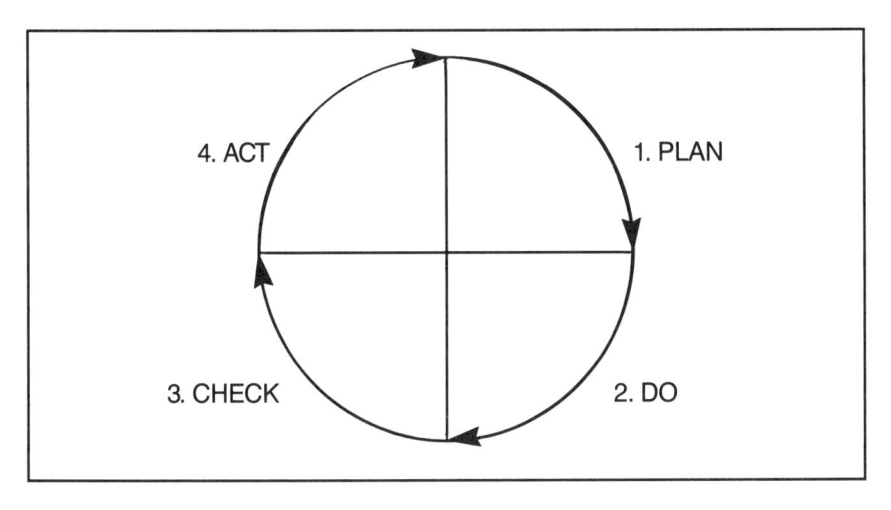

Figure 6.14 Shewhart-Deming cycle.

Plan, Do, Check, Act

Plan

What does the team wish to achieve? What can the team afford to do? How will the team reach its goal? Who will be responsible for carrying out each part of the plan? Who will the team be accountable to? How will the team be held accountable?

These questions must be answered realistically at the beginning of any treatment plan. A treatment plan must begin with a description and diagnosis of the process which produced the health problem(s). A detailed flow diagram (Figure 6.15) establishes a relative frame of reference for the team's proposed process improvement actions. The control charts (Figure 6.16), which supplement their process description, help the team differentiate common cause and special cause variation.

The patient's lifestyle and psychological processes will influence the recovery process. Many patients can and will want to invest their spiritual activities as well. Therefore, it is impossible for the patient to delegate responsibility for recovery to his or her care givers. It is unreasonable for the team to spend as much money as it wants unless the patient is picking up the tab.

The customer, the party paying the bill, must have a say-so in how the team is to be held accountable. World Class Health Care customers understand the value of integrated care and prevention. They are buying the lowest total cost health care, not the cheapest, and they have a right

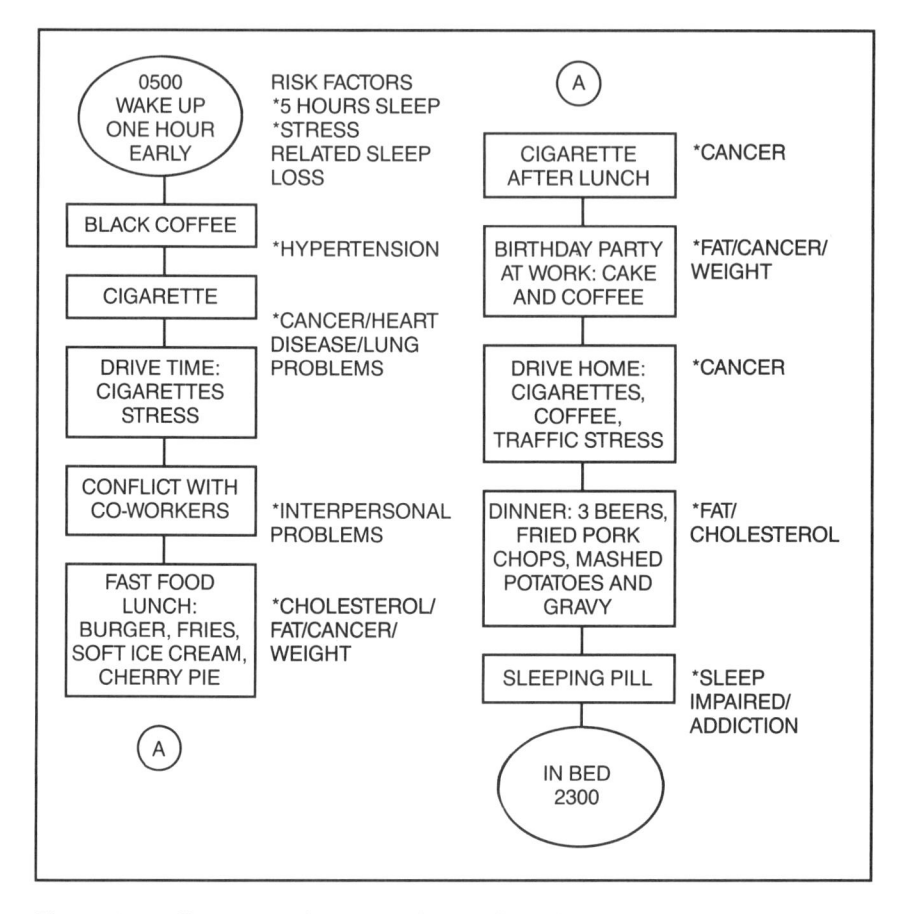

Figure 6.15 Summary of sample lifestyle flow diagram.

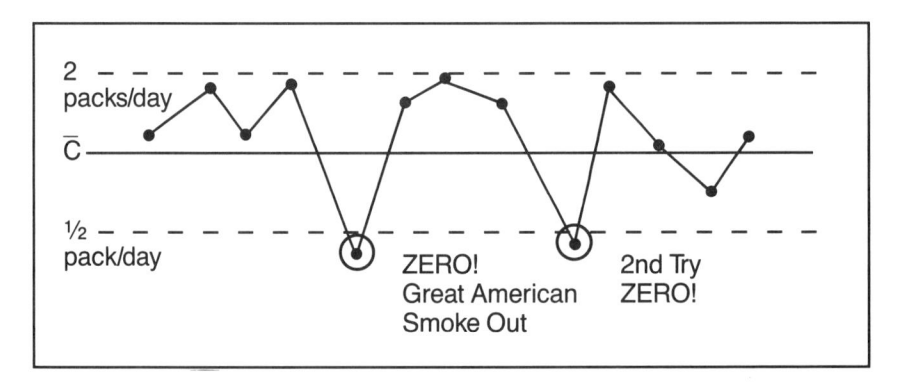

Figure 6.16 Control chart: number of cigarettes smoked per day. Control charts supplement lifestyle flow diagram.

to make sure quality care is delivered as promised.

Team goals must be specific. They must be defined clearly using language every team member understands. Goals must be measurable and results must be displayed so everyone can read them.

Health care goals must be process- as well as results-focused. The treatment process is as important as treatment outcomes, particularly for patients who have begun the process of dying. Health care goals must be flexible rather than rigid. As the team's knowledge expands, new quality of care choices become apparent.

Do

The Pareto principle (Figure 6.17) should be used in the same way a medical triage is used to prioritize an emergency treatment process. First things first.

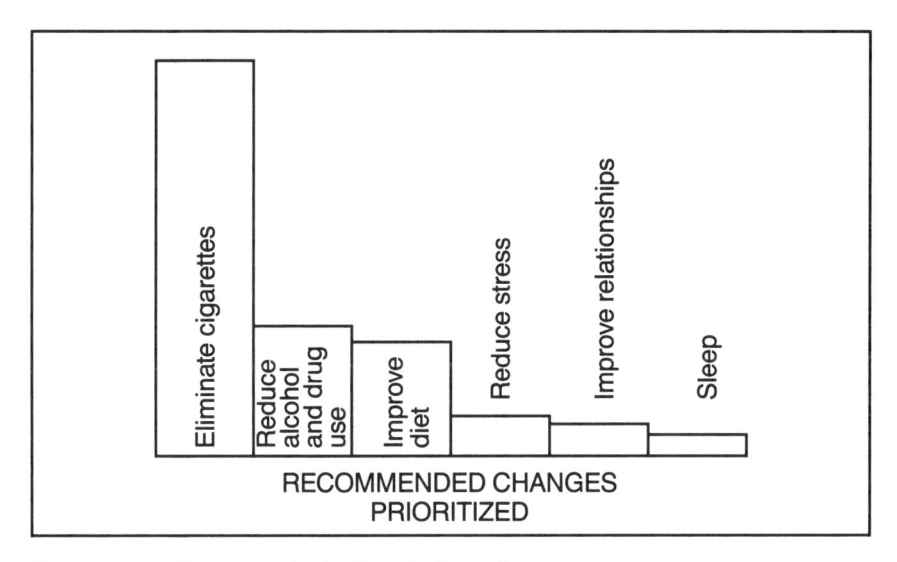

Figure 6.17 Pareto analysis lifestyle flow diagram.

If the patient enjoys good health, care can be focused on strengthening their level of well being. If the patient is seriously ill, physical and mental health problems must be addressed before the educational and lifestyle issues.

World Class Health Care treatment team members are actively involved team members. The treatment process is participatory.

Check

Everyone on the team must help with data collection and analysis. Data must be graphed over time using statistical charts. Medical doctors and their support personnel are best equipped to perform physical assessments. Mental health professionals are best prepared to do the requisite psychological assessments. Master-degreed therapists can work under the supervision of a qualified doctor to minimize expense. Nurse educators and patients are ideally suited for lifestyle assessments.

Physicians, behavioral science professionals, and nurse educators skilled in the use of process quality control methods must be key players in the delivery of quality health care. "Statistical thinking," as H. G. Wells observed, "will be as necessary for efficient citizenship as the ability to read and write."[14]

The statistical education of patients and care givers may prove to be the most powerful public health care policy strategy of this century. When everyone can speak the simple, common language of statistics, then society can move toward quality.

Act

Step four in the circular logic of the Shewhart-Deming cycle calls for continued action. Continued action must be guided by reliable, predictive tools. During this step in the cycle a new hypothesis must be proposed about how the team can process the knowledge it has gained. This knowledge guides the reasoned action the team will take to hold and improve the gains it has made.

Therapy, education, and statistical process control are the World Class Health Care tools of choice. Each tool can be used to raise the quality of care, reduce the costs of care, and hold gains made in the continuous improvement process of health.

Medical Cost Offset Effect

When people access comprehensive mental health services, demand for medical and surgical services decreases by up to 72 percent.[15] Because this decrease in demand can significantly reduce net medical costs, the phenomenon is called the *medical cost offset effect*. The body of evidence which confirms its existence has grown steadily over the past three decades. The evidence now grows by the day.

The cost offset effect was first noticed within the confines of a California-based health maintenance organization, Kaiser Permanente. Kaiser is a health maintenance organization which benefits financially from controlling costs.

A psychologist and a psychiatrist summarized their observations at

Kaiser in 1967; a single visit for psychotherapy reduced medical utilization by 60 percent over the following five years. Two to eight psychotherapy sessions reduced utilization by 75 percent over the following five years.[16, 17, 18]

This miraculous offset effect and the others which have been observed and recorded since were achieved accidentally. As people and health care purchasers decide to actively reduce their health care costs the effect will be seen more frequently and on purpose.

A 1984 meta-analysis of 58 controlled studies and analysis of the claim files for the Blue Cross/Blue Shield Federal Employees plan for 1974–1978 is one case in point. Forty-nine of the 58 reviewed studies reported significant decreases in medical service usage following mental health treatment.[15]

A report which reviewed Aetna's Federal Employees Health Benefits Program from 1980 through 1983 is another recent illustration of the power mental health services have to reduce total health care costs. A total of 26,915 families with at least one member receiving mental health services were compared to 16,468 families with no members receiving mental health services. Families who received mental health care experienced 36 consecutive months of decreasing health care costs. It is important to keep in mind these savings were achieved well in advance of the DRG prospective payment system.[18]

A civilian might assume psychologists, social workers, and other mental health professionals would applaud these findings. This is not necessarily the case. Many psychologists do not believe in the offset theory. The false precepts of archaic beliefs have trapped these professions with the same snare that holds the rest of us. Our system often pays psychiatrists, psychologists, and counselors to be voyeurs. They earn their fees not by bringing about solutions, but by investigating problems.

From the Freudian therapist's point of view a patient's simple need to feel well is not enough. Their a priori assumption is that a patient's character must be analyzed and reconstructed. Since this nebulous goal is impossible to quantify or define, theoretical (traditional) therapy can legitimately be unending. The therapist's privately held truths are forever shrouded in mystery.

A therapy which produces satisfactory results in eight to 10 visits is unwelcome. Unless therapists are prepared to do a volume business it is an economic threat. A brief therapy model which suggests five, one-hour visits are sufficient to resolve almost every complaint is ignored. When it cannot be ignored it is ridiculed.

The Brief Family Therapy Center in Wisconsin and the Brief Therapy Center of the Mental Research Institute in Palo Alto, California, are the traditional therapist's worst nightmares come true. The experience of these two brief therapy model clinics suggests therapeutic treatment and clinical solutions for depression, anxiety, alcoholism, and even cocaine addiction need not be connected to the core, underlying reasons for a mental health or addiction problem.

According to these two models, therapy need only investigate and create solutions to the problem. When the problem is resolved to the client's satisfaction, not the therapist's, therapy abruptly ends. Good therapy outcomes are routinely achieved in one to five visits by following Steve deShazer's[19] Brief therapy's Central Map (Figure 6.18).

Steve deShazer's therapy flow diagram is powerful in its simplicity.* According to deShazer,[20] "It emphasizes cooperation and builds on what the client is already doing. It avoids a need for them to resist the therapist's ideas."

Brief therapy is not a shortened version of the same old speculative theory. Brief therapy is science. deShazer bases his model on an understanding of variation. He uses empirical observation and inductive reasoning. His process improvement tasks are worthy of Shewhart.

A client who visits the Brief Family Therapy Center in Milwaukee is classified as either a "visitor," a "complainant," or a "customer." "Visitors" come through the coercion of a court order or peer pressure. "Complainants" bring their complaints. Complaints, according to deShazer, are a result of chance. In his words, "Their problems are just damn bad luck." "Customers" are those people who want to do something about their complaints.

Brief therapy begins when a person calls to schedule an appointment. Each potential customer is asked to collect data by observing their problem. During the first session the therapist helps the visitor or complainant focus on their complaint. Together they produce a precise operational definition of the exact problem to be solved. They outline the process(es) and sequence of events which are causing the complaints. The knowledge and insight gained from this first session can quickly turn a visitor or a complainant into a customer.

The therapist and customer then conduct a mutual search for exceptions in the process. Are there special causes? Are there times when things are better? The therapist works with the customer to establish specific therapy goals by asking, "How will you know when the problem is resolved? Specifically, if a miracle occurred and the problem disappeared, what would be different?" When this goal is achieved, both the customer and therapist will know therapy has ended.

Customers make rapid progress by trying solutions they help construct. Brief therapy solutions invariably amount to "doing something different." Doing something different, which sometimes means thinking something different, disturbs the pattern which maintains the complaint. Desirable special causes are repeated and built into the customer's daily lifestyle process. A new process replaces the old process.

---

*Therapy differs from psychotherapy. Psychotherapy implies the clinician is dealing with the psyche, a theoretical entity. Since therapists focus their attention on context the use of the word psychotherapy is inappropriate.

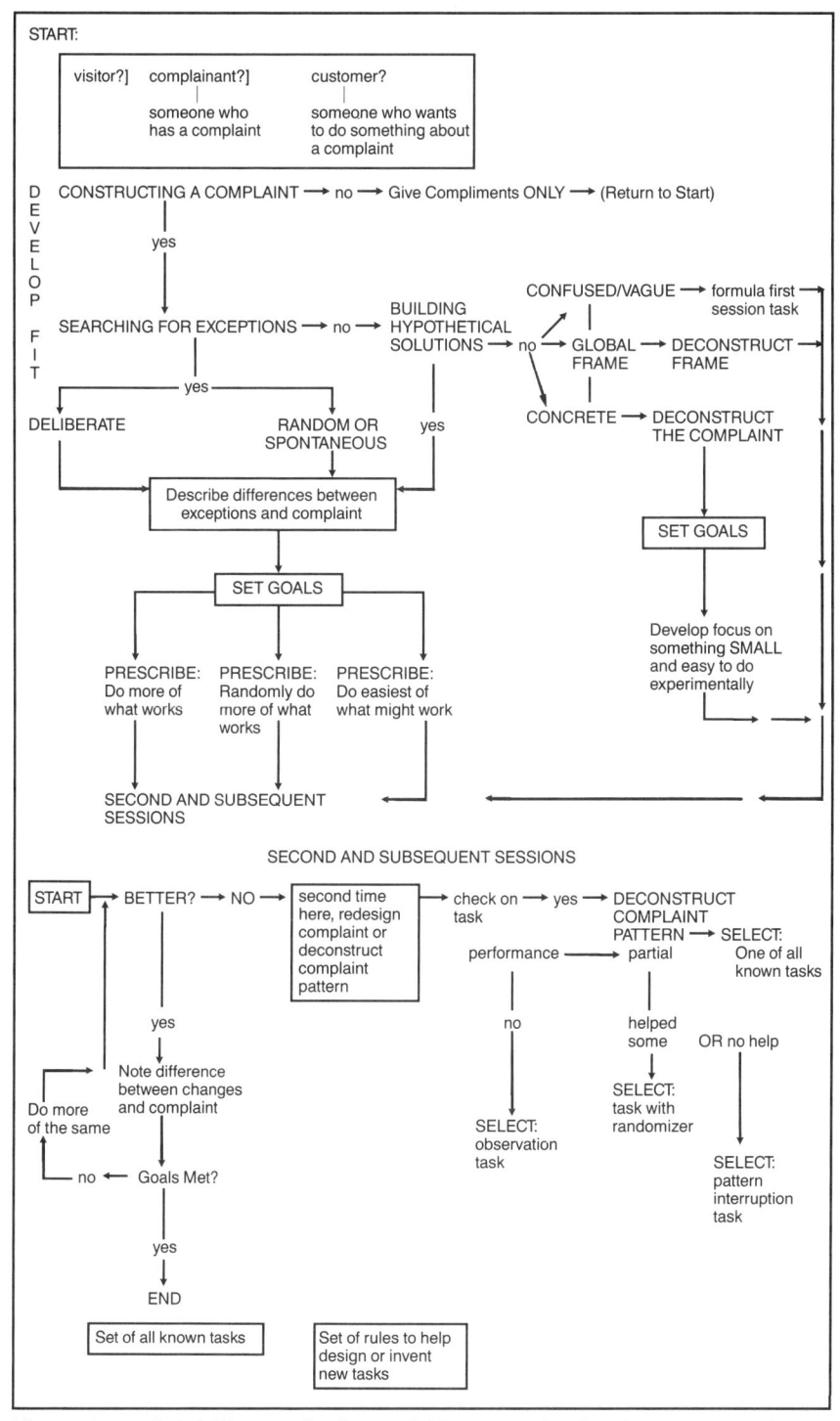

Figure 6.18 Brief Therapy's Central Map standardized process reduces variation between therapists. *Used with permission of W.W. Norton and Company. Steve de Shazer,* Clues, Investigating Solutions in Brief Therapy, *page 86.*

Visualize a brief therapy case study as an exercise in statistical process control. For instance, a customer arrives with a complaint; he, a former high school wrestler, picks saloon fights several nights a week and he is suffering from some dicey legal problems. He would like to stop but he claims this behavior is beyond his control. He averages two to four fights per week. During the course of the first session the therapist and client discover an exception to this pattern. He never fights on the days that he runs more than two miles.

The therapist asks the complainant, "On a scale from one to 10 how much chance do you give yourself that this problem can be solved?" The complainant answers, "An eight."

The therapist expresses his mutual optimism and leaves the young man for five minutes to consult with the therapy team behind the mirror. The customer is left alone with his thoughts.

When the therapist returns he offers the team's compliments to the customer for his insight. He is congratulated for the hard work he has already done in trying to solve the problem. He is praised for confronting the problem. He is praised for keeping his appointment. He is told that the team thinks he should run two and a half miles every day to see if it works.

On the following session the customer shares his improvement with pride. On the days he runs no fights have occurred. Even when he doesn't run, fights are down 40 percent and the urge to fight is diminished. The therapist asks, "On a scale of one to 10, how hopeful are you that this problem can be solved?" The customer answers, "A 10."

The therapist leaves him alone to consult with the team behind the mirror. The therapist returns to offer the team's compliments. He worked hard on the task. He looks proud of himself and he should be. The team also gives his chances of solving the problem a 10.

Therapy ends during the third and final session. The customer says he is up to three miles a day. He has not even experienced any urge to pick a fight. This is the first time in five years he has gone for three weeks with no barroom brawls. There is no need for a theoretical rehashing or analysis of the old problem. It is gone. The illustration (Figure 6.19) shows how his behavior was controlled, in Shewhart's sense of the word, by repeating a desirable special cause.

Therapy sessions are observed and videotaped by other therapists from behind a one-way mirror. The therapist leaves the client alone to think for at least five minutes each session. During this time the therapist consults with the team behind the mirror. When the therapist returns he compliments the customer on his or her good work and recommends trying more of the solution which is known to work. If no exceptions (special causes) are known, the customer and therapist construct a solution the customer thinks might work and he is assigned that as a task. The mirror and standardized team approach ensure consistent, quality therapy.

Brief therapy can resolve attitude, emotional, and addiction problems in

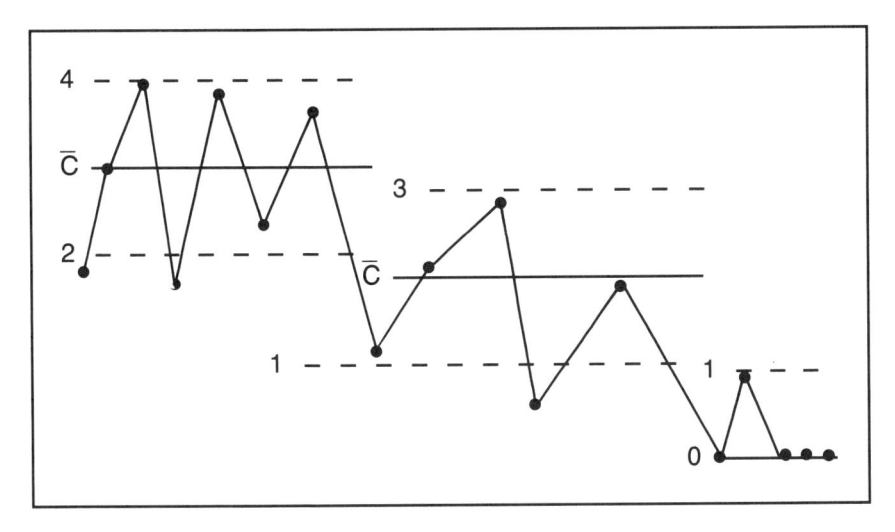

Figure 6.19 A behavior was controlled, in Shewhart's sense of the word, by including a desirable special cause in the behavior process.

only a few visits. It is a scientific process (hypothesis, experiment, test hypothesis) which can be replicated. Brief therapy results are public truths which can be tested and verified with empirical data. Brief therapy holds great promise for World Class Health Care. It is a key which can help us reduce the overuse of medical, surgical, hospital, and traditional mental health services.

Education

People have an infinite capacity to learn. New learning occurs every day. Learned habits are practiced every hour. Practiced habits are the rhythm of life.

What is healthy and what is unhealthy is a less dominant influence on this rhythm than which behaviors are reinforced or rewarded, and which are ignored or punished. There are two ways to reinforce learning.

One way is to link the reward directly to behavior. For example a gambler hits the jackpot every time he pulls the handle on a one-armed bandit. This reinforcement schedule is called a frequency ratio.

The other way is to link the reward to a time factor. Weekly paychecks are a good example. This reinforcement schedule is called a frequency interval.

The frequency ratio and the frequency interval may be fixed (it occurs every time or every set number of times a behavior is exhibited) or variable (it happens on a random basis). The manner in which these two reinforcement schedules are combined creates a relationship between behavior and reward. The relationship determines how long a learned behavior will last.

The quickest way to teach someone to do something is to reward him or her every time he or she does what you want done. When the reward is subsequently withheld, this type of learning is rapidly extinguished. The illustration (Figure 6.20) summarizes the behavior curves associated with each type of reward.

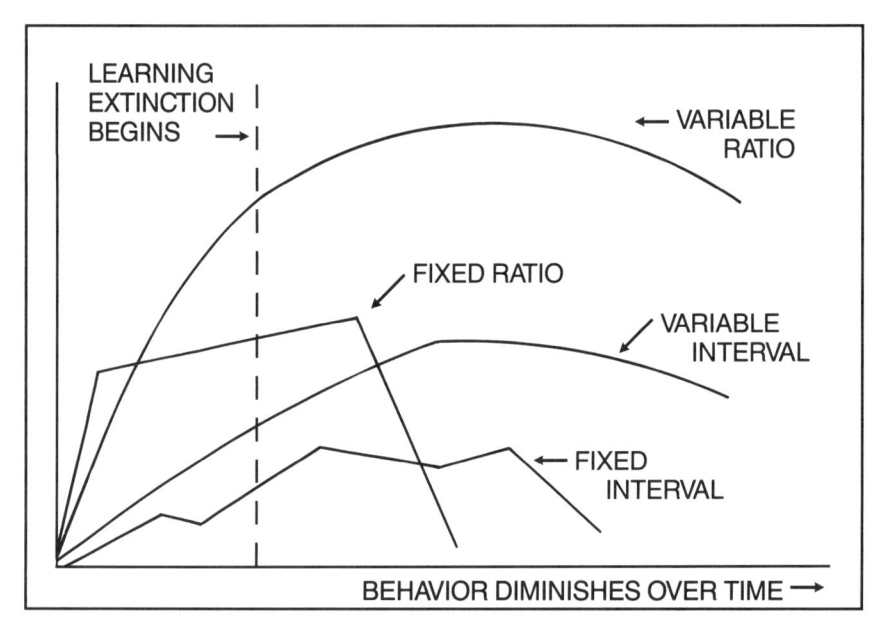

Figure 6.20 Behavior curves associated with each type of reward: variable ratio, fixed ratio, variable interval, and fixed interval.

Health habit behaviors tend to be on the other end of the learning scale. They are rewarded randomly with variable ratios and at variable intervals. They take time and circumstance to learn. Once learned and internalized they are difficult to modify. Even an intermittent reinforcement serves to sustain the behavior.

A lifetime cigarette smoker occasionally can live into his nineties. An alcoholic or chemically dependent person can inexplicably die of old age. Every so often a newborn baby is saved by a liver transplant. Once in a blue moon an 85-year-old man testifies to the benefits of dialysis.

These infrequent, against-the-odds victories reward the system and people vicariously. These are the variable ratio and variable interval success stories which reinforce old medical beliefs. They make us root for the underdog. They help us rationalize self-destructive lifestyles. They sustain and nurture our superstitious belief in life's forgiving nature and medicine's ability to rescue dying people. The mechanical advantage medical technology can gain on our hearts, lungs, and livers is no match for the power of good health habits.

Health habits rarely change by accident. They can be improved on purpose. Scores of well-designed health education classes have demonstrated education's ability to motivate people. Health habits can be profoundly changed for the better following a workshop which lasts no more than three hours.[21]

Routine lifestyle assessments and interventions done by trained nurse educators are an invaluable addition to an integrated treatment plan. Predictable hospitalizations related to predictable disease dictate the core curriculum.

How to stop smoking
How to end drug and alcohol misuse and abuse
How to balance emotions
How to maintain an ideal weight
How to make life and death decisions with dignity
How to stay physically fit

Health education classes create a supportive environment for change. A supportive environment is important to personal growth. The fellowship of Alcoholics Anonymous testifies to that fact. Volunteer support groups like AA, Gamblers Anonymous, Overeaters Anonymous, and Weight Watchers can make a marvelous contribution to a person's health and well being. Self-help groups can and do help people quit smoking. They can and do help people cope with terminal disease. They can and do help people work through the grief which accompanies the process of death and dying. They can do even more in the future.

Self-help groups create a feeling of belonging for members. The need to belong motivates. Membership benefits include friendly competition, peer pressure, and structured activities in a safe environment.

It is poor form to drink at an AA meeting or to eat a box of chocolates during an Overeaters Anonymous meeting, so these events rarely occur. Time spent in safety means less time is available to misbehave.

Members learn how to help themselves. They learn how to help others. Both activities are rewarding. The group recognizes the personal expertise each member has with a problem the group shares. Their expertise is put to good use. Group members find respect. They experience a sense of accomplishment. They find a sense of self-esteem. Self-respect and self-esteem are potent forces for change in anyone's life.

People are almost as predictable as hospitalizations. When a new behavior is more rewarding than an old behavior, the new behavior, and the thinking which goes with it, wins out. Education backed by economic incentives, financial penalties, and support groups can improve health habits enough to minimize the demand for expensive, hospital-based services.

Even in the absence of a big stick or a tempting carrot on a stick, health education in the physician's office has proven it can reduce a person's risk for accidental injury, cardiovascular disease, and cancer. The *INSURE* project, sponsored by 88 insurance companies and a host of foundations, studied 4,218 people. Half were adults and half were children. Their seven-year Lifecycle Preventive Health Services project cost a modest $1.7 million.

Reduced cigarette smoking, increased exercise, and more frequent use of seat belts were noted. Woman who received health education counseling did breast self-examinations more frequently. *INSURE* investors concluded health education had earned them a good return.

When education is combined with the medical and behavioral sciences it can earn our nation an even better return—quality health care at affordable prices.

Process Quality Control

Statistical thinking and the tools of process quality control are as indispensable to quality health care as they are to quality manufacturing. The central element of statistical process control is the central element to quality health care, brainpower. World Class brainpower runs on clear thinking and statistical reasoning.

Brainpower, used from the perspective of process quality control, is distinguished by four quality characteristics.

1. Process quality control emphasizes prevention.
2. Process quality control graphs data, in sequence over time so decisions are based on fact, not someone's memory.
3. Process quality control creates a scientific environment where experimental design, data collection technique, and analytic methods constantly improve.
4. Process quality control charts graphically predict the capacity a process has for producing a desired result.

Quality control involves taking action for the purpose of achieving a desired end. The desired end of quality health care from the viewpoint of process quality control is resilient good health.

World Class Health Care is a radical departure from existing health care delivery system models. Hospitals, clinics, health maintenance organizations, and even holistic medicine place medical knowledge, political power, and economic clout under physician control.

Medical record data are recorded in an incomprehensible language. Medical records and the knowledge they can impart are kept under lock and key. They are concealed from the patient even though the patient is the person who ultimately controls and must live with treatment process outcomes.

World Class Health Care empowers patients with knowledge, and the statistical tools of process quality control. All members of the World Class Health Care team—patient, physician, psychologist, and nurse educator—have equal access to the data contained in the medical record.

Medical record data are graphed using check sheets, histograms, Pareto charts, scattergrams, cause-and-effect diagrams, run charts, control charts, and flow diagrams. Thus, the medical record is written in a "picture" language every patient and care giver can understand and use.

Check sheets, histograms, and Pareto charts (Figure 6.21) graphically portray the impact of problems on health status. These charts enable care givers to concentrate on the vital few factors which cause disease.

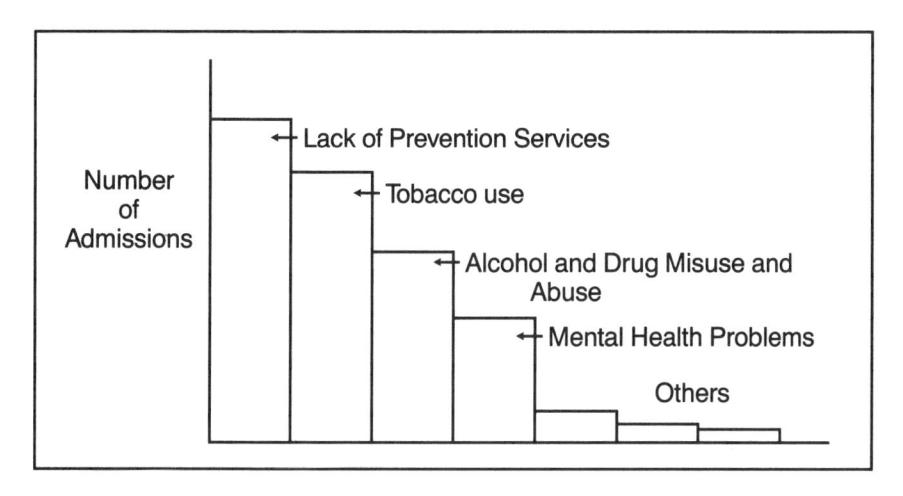

Figure 6.21 Pareto chart rank orders routine causes of hospitalization.

The cause-and-effect diagram (Figure 6.22), also known as an Ishikawa or fishbone diagram,[22] organizes ideas as to which causes can produce the desired effect, resilient good health.

Run charts can be used to identify trends. Control charts set upper and lower control limits for normal variations in health status. For example, under the traditional medical model a college student finds her diabetic roommate semicomatose. She calls 911 to the rescue. The following bills are generated:

Ambulance run	$750
Critical care emergency room charges	800
Intensive care unit admission	3,000
Medical ward admission	600
Lab, including blood gases and STAT work	1,000
Chest X-ray	120
Pharmacy	520
Private physician fee	500
	$7,290

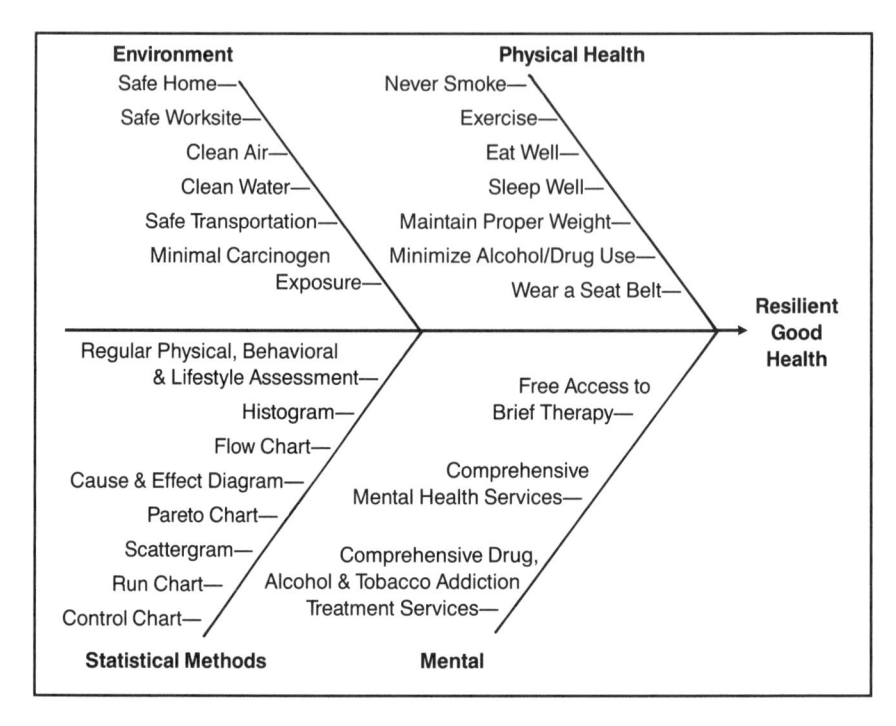

```
                Environment                    Physical Health
            Safe Home—\              Never Smoke—\
            Safe Worksite—\          Exercise—\
              Clean Air—\            Eat Well—\
              Clean Water—\          Sleep Well—\
          Safe Transportation—\      Maintain Proper Weight—\
          Minimal Carcinogen         Minimize Alcohol/Drug Use—\
              Exposure—\             Wear a Seat Belt—\
                                                             → Resilient
                                                               Good
                                                               Health
    Regular Physical, Behavioral
      & Lifestyle Assessment—         Free Access to
              Histogram—/             Brief Therapy—\
              Flow Chart—/
     Cause & Effect Diagram—/         Comprehensive
              Pareto Chart—/       Mental Health Services—\
              Scattergram—/
              Run Chart—/          Comprehensive Drug,
              Control Chart—/    Alcohol & Tobacco Addiction
                                    Treatment Services—/
          Statistical Methods             Mental
```

Figure 6.22 The Ishikawa[22] or fishbone diagram shows cause and effect.

In a World Class Health Care system the fragile diabetic plots her blood sugar level on a control chart (Figure 6.23) two times each day. This routine was established when she was young and she is familiar with her blood sugar patterns.

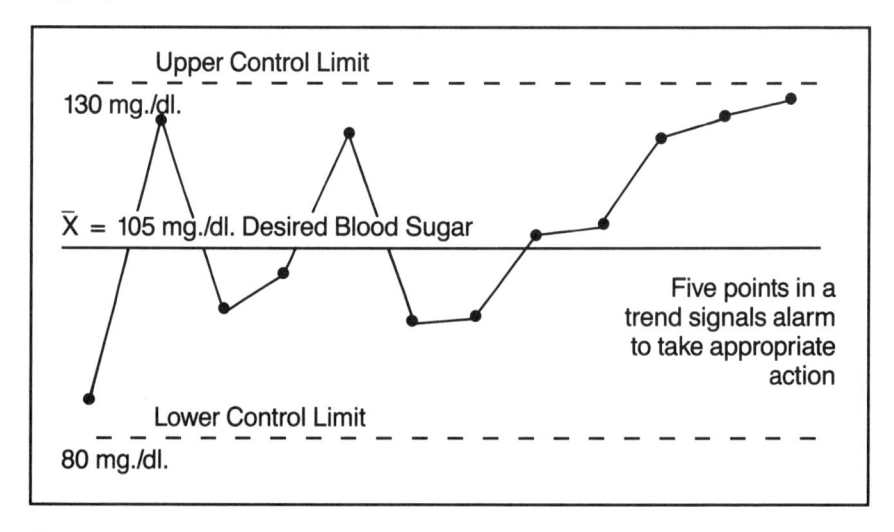

```
         Upper Control Limit
    ─ ─ ─ ─ ─ ─ ─ ─ ─ ─ ─ ─ ─ ─ ─ ─ ─ ─
    130 mg./dl.

    X̄ = 105 mg./dl. Desired Blood Sugar
    ─────────────────────────────────────
                              Five points in a
                              trend signals alarm
                              to take appropriate
                              action
         Lower Control Limit
    ─ ─ ─ ─ ─ ─ ─ ─ ─ ─ ─ ─ ─ ─ ─ ─ ─ ─
    80 mg./dl.
```

Figure 6.23 Diabetic control chart.

On the sixth data point of this chart she noted, "I think I am getting the flu." On the eighth point she wrote, "Vomited three times. Can't eat. Skipped insulin." On the twelfth point, the sixth in a trend, she telephoned her nurse educator, a diabetologist.

After a brief assessment, her educator placed her on a sliding scale regime of regular insulin coupled with strict control chart monitoring four times a day. The following charge was generated:

One telephone consultation $18.00

World Class Health Care reduced the cost of a single crisis by $7,272.

Blood pressure readings can be charted for those with hypertension. Potassium levels can be charted to monitor anorexic individuals. Drinking can be charted for alcoholics. Anginal pain frequency can be tracked for heart attack victims. The opportunities to observe variation by graphing data are infinite.

In all cases the upper control limit and the lower control limit of a chosen quality characteristic are restricted to harmless variation. Life-threatening variations, those requiring hospitalization, can be minimized or eliminated.

Reducing variation is an infinite process and therefore lends itself to continuous improvement. The integrated treatment team expects an ever-increasing quality of care and ever-decreasing cost of care.

Scatter diagrams like the one in Figure 6.24 can be used to display the relationship between two variables. Flow diagrams like deShazer's[19] Central Map (Figure 6.18) can be used to detail all the steps in the health status process.

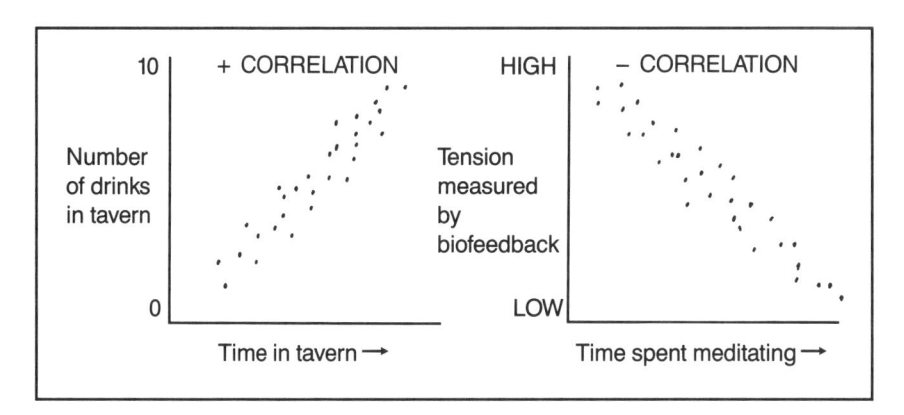

Figure 6.24 A scatter diagram displaying the relationship between two variables.

Shewhart illustrated a practical quality report format in the final pages of the *Economic Control of Quality of Manufactured Product*.[4] His model played an important role in the international World Class Manufacturing revolution. In time it will revolutionize the medical record format.

Shewhart said a quality report should do two things:

1. Indicate the presence of assignable causes of variation in each of the quality characteristics.
2. Indicate the seriousness of the trouble and the steps taken to eliminate it.

A World Class Health Care approach would use the following tools: a physical assessment, control charts, a Michigan Alcoholism Screening Test, and a Beck Depression Inventory (Figures 6.25 and 6.26; Table 6.1). The medical record face sheet for Brenda, the suicide victim in our melodrama, would have looked like this:

Brenda_____: Quality Characteristics: (a) Blood pressure (b) weight (c) self-medication with alcohol (d) self-report depression scale 1–10 established following Beck's Depression Scale Inventory results* (e) suicidal ideation.

A World Class Health Care treatment team would have collected data on Brenda's mental health and lifestyle status far in advance of her pregnancy. Her previous history of suicidal thinking and her habitual use of alcohol would have sent out warning signals to the treatment team before an amniocentesis study was done. The study's report would have been shared in a supportive, safe, and routine team conference setting. A brief hospital stay following the conference would have prevented the suicide.

Statistical process tools and teamwork transfer considerable power from the lone physician to the patient and the integrated treatment team. The entire team, including the patient, becomes an integral part of a hospital's medical staff. This collegial relationship is crucially important to quality health care.

In conclusion, the integrated treatment team using the statistical tools of process quality control changes *everything* about the way health care is delivered for the better.

As the new delivery system replaces the old one C. I. Lewis[2] offers comforting words:

> Any contradiction between the old truth and the new is verbal only, because the old word "disease" has a new meaning. The old word is retained but the old concept is discarded as a poor intellectual instrument and replaced by a better one.

---

*For commentary on the consequence of self-reported depression see Wells, Stewart, Hayes, et al, JAMA, August 18, 1989, Vol. 262, No. 7: 914–919.

QUALITY CONTROL REPORT

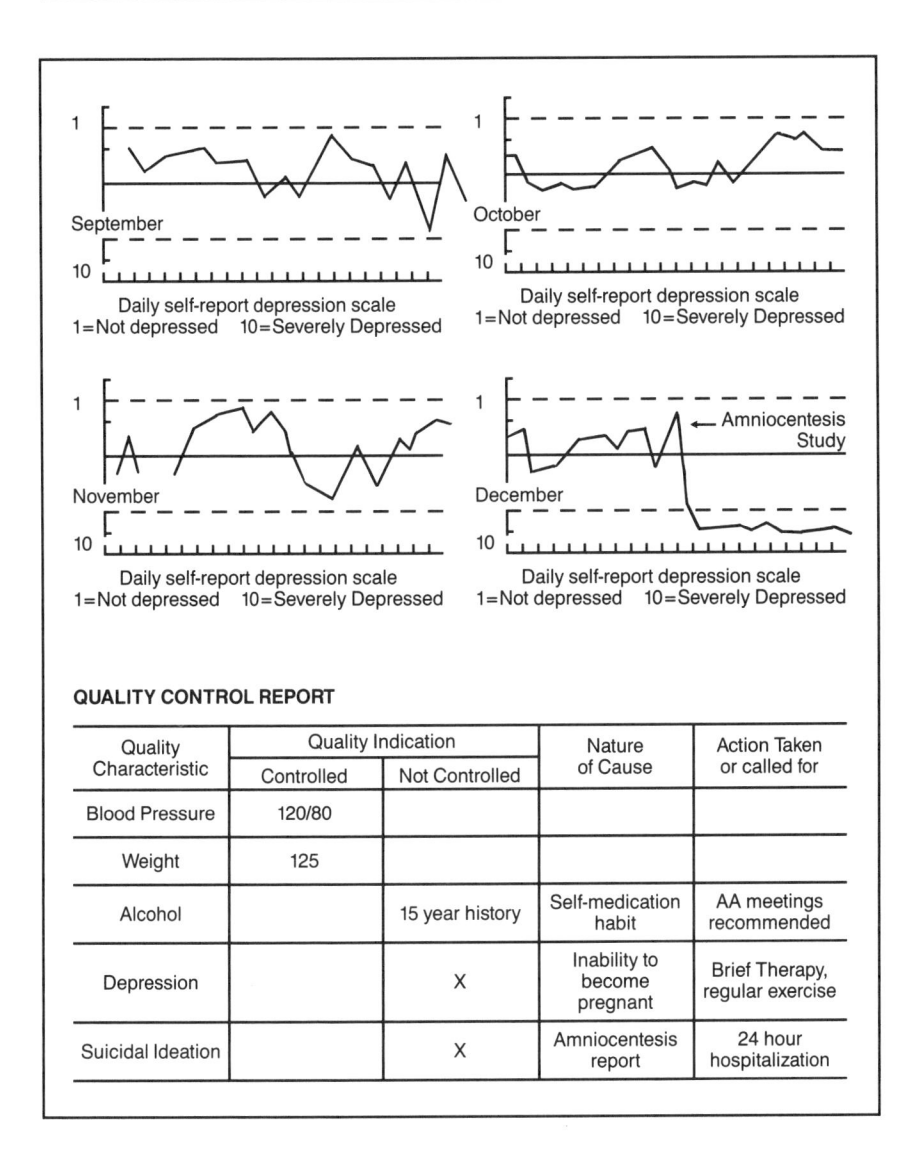

Quality Characteristic	Quality Indication		Nature of Cause	Action Taken or called for
	Controlled	Not Controlled		
Blood Pressure	120/80			
Weight	125			
Alcohol		15 year history	Self-medication habit	AA meetings recommended
Depression		X	Inability to become pregnant	Brief Therapy, regular exercise
Suicidal Ideation		X	Amniocentesis report	24 hour hospitalization

Figure 6.25 World class health care medical record face sheet sample. *Adapted with permission of the American Society for Quality Control. Walter Shewhart,* Economic Control of Quality of Manufactured Product, *pages 420-421.*

MICHIGAN ALCOHOLISM SCREENING TEST

NAME: BRENDA _____

DATE: _____

1. Do you feel you are a normal drinker?	No **(Yes)**
2. Have you ever awakened in the morning after some drinking the night before and found that you could not remember part of the evening?	**(Yes)** No
3. Does your wife (or husband or parents) ever worry or complain about your drinking?	**(Yes)** No
4. Can you stop drinking without a struggle after one or two drinks?	No **(Yes)**
5. Do you ever feel badly about drinking?	**(Yes)** No
6. Do you ever try to limit your drinking to certain times of the day or to certain places?	**(Yes)** No
7. Do your friends and relatives think that you are a normal drinker?	No **(Yes)**
8. Are you always able to stop when you want to?	No **(Yes)**
9. Have you ever attended a meeting of Alcoholics Anonymous?	Yes **(No)**
10. Have you gotten into fights when drinking?	Yes **(No)**
11. Has drinking ever created problems with you and your wife (husband)?	**(Yes)** No
12. Has your wife (husband or family member) ever gone to anyone for help about your drinking?	Yes **(No)**
13. Have you ever lost friends or girlfriends/boyfriends because of drinking?	Yes **(No)**
14. Have you ever gotten into trouble at work because of drinking?	Yes **(No)**
15. Have you ever lost a job because of drinking?	Yes **(No)**
16. Have you ever neglected your obligations, your family or your work for two days or more in a row because of drinking?	Yes **(No)**
17. Do you ever drink before noon?	Yes **(No)**
18. Have you ever been told you have liver trouble?	Yes **(No)**
19. Have you ever had DI's (delirium tremens), severe shaking, heard voices or seen things that weren't there after heavy drinking?	Yes **(No)**
20. Have you ever gone to anyone for help about your drinking?	Yes **(No)**
21. Have you ever been in a hospital because of drinking?	Yes **(No)**
22. Have you ever been a patient in a psychiatric hospital or on a psychiatric ward of a general hospital where drinking was part of the problem?	Yes **(No)**
23. Have you ever been seen at a psychiatric or mental health clinic or gone to a doctor, or clergyman for help with an emotional problem in which drinking has played a part?	Yes **(No)**
24. Have you ever been arrested, even for a few hours because of drunken behavior?	**(Yes)** No
25. Have you ever been arrested for drunk driving or driving after drinking?	**(Yes)** No

Figure 6.26 Michigan Alcoholism Screening test.
Used with permission of M.L. Selzer, MD.

> **BECK DEPRESSION INVENTORY***
> **Sample Questions**
>
> Choose one statement under each letter that best describes you for the last 30 days. Circle the number to the left of the statement you have chosen.
>
> F. 0 I don't feel I am being punished.
>   1 I feel I may be punished.
>   2 I expect to be punished.
>   3 I feel I am being punished.
>
> I. 0 I don't have any thoughts of killing myself.
>   1 I have thoughts of killing myself, but I would not carry them out.
>   2 I would like to kill myself.
>   3 I would kill myself if I had the chance.
>
> *Reprinted with permission from the Psychological Corporation.
>
> From the Beck Depression Inventory. Copyright © 1987 by Aaron T. Beck, M.D. Reproduced by permission of publisher, The Psychological Corporation, San Antonio, Texas. All rights reserved.

Table 6.1 Beck Depression Inventory.

REFERENCES

1. Kuhn, T.S. *The Structure of Scientific Revolutions.* Chicago: University of Chicago Press, 1970.

2. Lewis, C.I. *Mind and the World Order: Outline of a Theory of Knowledge.* New York: Dover Press, 1929.

3. Einstein, A. *Relativity.* New York: Crown Publishers, 1916.

4. Shewhart, W.A. *Economic Control of Quality of Manufactured Product.* New York: MacMillan and Van Nostrand, 1931. Commemorative reissue Milwaukee: ASQC Quality Press, 1980.

5. Shewhart, W.A. *Statistical Method from the Viewpoint of Quality Control.* New York: Dover Publications, 1939.

6. Deming, W.E. *Out of the Crisis.* Cambridge: Massachusetts Institute of Technology, 1988.

7. Masaaki, I. *Kaizen.* New York: Random House, 1986.

8. Juran, J.M. *Juran's Quality Control Handbook,* 4th ed. New York: McGraw-Hill, 1988.

9. Commisson on Professional and Hospital Activities. *International Classification of Diseases,* 9th revision, Clinical Modification. Ann Arbor, MI: Edwards Brothers, 1978.

10. *Diagnostic and Statistical Manual of Mental Disorders,* 3rd Edition, Revised. Washington, DC: American Psychiatric Association.

11. Surgeon General. *Healthy People: Surgeon General's Report on Health Promotion and Disease Prevention.* Washington, DC: GPO, 1979.

12. Amler, R.W., and H.B. Dull. *Closing the Gap.* New York: Oxford Press, 1987.

13. Thorndike, E.L. See Hilgard, E.R., and Bower, G.H. *Theories of Learning,* Century Psychology Series, Appleton Century Crafts, New York, 1966.

14. Scherkenbach, W.W. *The Deming Route to Quality and Productivity: Road Maps and Road Blocks.* Washington, DC: CEEP Press Books, 1988.

15. Mumford, E., H.J. Shlesinger, and G.V. Glass. "A New Look at Evidence About Reduced Cost of Medical Utilization Following Mental Health Treatment." *American Journal of Psychiatry* 141, No. 10 (1984): 1145-1158.

16. Follette, W.T., and N.A. Cummings. "Psychiatric Services and Medical Utilization in a Prepaid Health Plan Setting: Part I." *Medical Care* Jan-Feb (1967) 5 No. 1: 25-35.

17. Cummings, N.A., and W.T. Follette. "Psychiatric Services and Medical Utilization in a Prepaid Health Plan Setting, Part II." *Medical Care* 6, No. 1 (Jan-Feb 1968): 31-41.

18. Cummings, N.A. "Prolonged (Ideal) Versus Short-Term (Realistic) Psychotherapy." *Professional Psychology* (November 1977): 491-501.

19. Holder, H.D., and J.O. Blose. "Changes in Healthcare Costs and Utilization Associated with Mental Health Treatment." *Hospital Community Psychiatry* 38, No. 10 (1987): 1070-75.

20. deShazer, S. *Clues—Investigating Solutions in Brief Therapy.* New York: W.W. Norton and Company, 1988.

21. deShazer, S. "A Requiem for Power." *Contemporary Family Therapy* (Summer 1988): 69-76.

22. *Positive Pulse.* A program to promote healthy lifestyles. United General Hospital, Sedro-Woolley, WA, 1985.

23. Ishikawa, K. "What Is Total Quality Control?" In *Quality Control Handbook* edited by K. Ishikawa. Englewood Cliffs, NJ: Prentice-Hall, 1985.

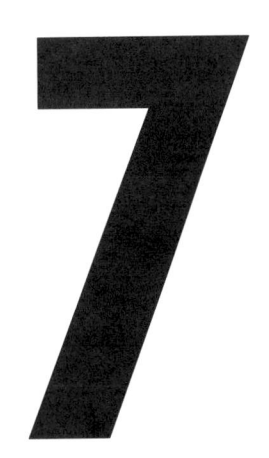

QUALITY INITIATIVES

> A society is no better than the quality of the people it produces.
> Eric Trist[1]
> *The Evolution of Socio-Technical Systems*

Self-preservation and self-interest have already created hairline fractures in traditional conceptual boundaries. The costs of keeping its shell intact will soon be prohibitive. The spectacular inefficiency and waste of our present health care system can and must be eliminated. Once we replace our outdated beliefs with a World Class Health Care philosophy the expense of health care will avalanche. Access to care can be assured for all citizens. The quality initiatives, clear thinking, and statistical reasoning can be made at any time and any place in the World Class Health Care process. We can control our health care future.

The World Class Health Care process includes raw materials (health status) and customer reaction (resilient good health). The quality of health and lifestyle a patient maintains prior to the presentation of a complaint or symptom predetermines the outcome and expense of every treatment. Any person requiring hospitalization necessarily must accept substantial responsibility for both. The patient is, after all, his own customer. In the jargon of quality control engineers, the medical arts process is his next customer.

Malpractice cases which involve lifestyle and self-inflicted diseases will be deemed frivolous long before World Class Health Care is legislated into our judicial system. Plaintiffs and lawyers who persist in pressing these cases upon the courts will be held in contempt. Malicious intent or a gross misjudgment based on obsolete diagnosis and treatment protocols will be the only legitimate grounds for a lawsuit.

World Class Health Care will transform our litigious society into a culture which values quality for quality's sake. One day, our culture will be one in which individuals voluntarily assume personal responsibility for the continuous improvement of quality health care.

Quality initiatives can be made in any and every social structure segment. Individuals, families, employers, and our government can all make meaningful contributions to the cause.

Individual Initiative

Seven common sense health habits have withstood the test of time. Once an individual adopts them, good health becomes a habit. Omitting them creates an odds-on chance for an expensive encounter with the health care industry.

1. Never smoke.
2. Exercise regularly.
3. Minimize or eliminate the misuse and abuse of alcohol and drugs.
4. Get a good night's sleep every night.
5. Eat breakfast and maintain a low fat diet.
6. Maintain your proper weight.
7. Wear a seat belt when you are in a vehicle.

Good health is everything it is cracked up to be. If feels good. Feeling good is its own reward. Feeling good can overpower the inertia of poor health.

Poor health is a hard habit to break but it can be done. The rewards of a satisfying cigarette, a routine afternoon cocktail, or an unsafe sexual encounter are mighty attractive to most people. They feel good, too.

How does a person know which good feeling to follow? Clear thinking, statistical reasoning, choice, and practice. Minimization, rationalization, and denial are booby-traps which can obliterate all four. They threaten us always. They work to separate us from our behavior, our attitudes, emotions, and the predictable consequences of a chosen lifestyle. They make us believe we are invincible. Defusing these bombs is a tricky business because the only way it can be done is to open ourselves up to others.

Opening up is forever a thorny task. It involves the real and imagined risks for embarrassment. We fear new knowledge. We are afraid of rejection. Medical doctors, psychologists, and nurse educators can help people avoid the errors of self-diagnosis, self-treatment, and independent introspection.

Family practitioners, their physician assistants, and nurse practitioners are exceptional resources for maintaining health. They know the limitations of medicine and they know its strengths. Their expertise is best used for education, immunizations, the treatment of routine infections, family planning, and sexual disease control. Their best technology is affordable. Many charge less than $10 to screen for high blood cholesterol, high blood pressure, diabetes, and cancer. A few provide these services for free. These contributions are invaluable to any person who wants to stay well. The person who wants to stay well must speak openly with them. Patients cannot expect to receive cost-effective, quality care when they force their care givers to play a lifestyle guessing game.

Physicians are an excellent referral resource for other specialists who treat psychological, emotional, educational, and chemical dependency problems. The importance of mental health cannot be overstated. The skills mental health professionals bring to health care are as important as education and medical technology.

Some doctors and their patients have learned to use trial and error to resolve the pressures of emotional distress. This approach to treatment is harmful. It is downright dangerous for people to suffer through addiction, emotional, and psychological distress without expert assistance.

Affordable, effective therapeutic approaches are available for the treatment of depression, anxiety, interpersonal problems, alcohol, and drug addiction. The statistical tools of process quality control can be used to chart trends and signal a warning of problems. As is the case with medicines, few current therapies are as efficient as they will be in the future; all are better than they have been in the past. All require skills which take considerable study to master. Luckily, the statistical process control tools required for health maintenance and improvement are easy to learn and use.

Taking a personal quality initiative to stay well requires a lifelong commitment to learning. Our bodies and our health care needs change as we age. The more a person knows about his health at any age, the better he is prepared to care for himself. Education empowers.

Quality education depends on good teachers and good books. Good health educators can be found in colleges, hospitals, and community service agencies. Good teachers have good credentials. They invite questions, encourage debate, and insist on class participation. Look for those characteristics in selecting your teachers.

Reading is a fundamental quality health skill. Convenience makes up for what reading lacks in the way of one-on-one guidance and the social support found in a classroom. With practice, reading becomes its own reward. New ideas and new information can be tried on for size. These three books are worth reading: (1) *The Social Transformation of American Medicine, The Rise of a Sovereign Industry*,[2] *Nutrition Concepts and Controversies*,[3] and *Aerobics*.[4]

Sooner or later educated, empowered people assume responsibility for their behavior and health. Under a World Class Health Care system educated people become champions of change. They are expected to empower others.

Well-educated consumers are assertive buyers. This is as it should be. Responsible consumerism can play the central role in establishing World Class Health Care status in the health care market.

It may be difficult to find World Class Health Care providers in the early 1990s. The best consumer tactic is to shop and shop hard for a provider who will meet your standards and expectations. Use the following checklist to screen potential providers.

	YES	NO
1. Does the provider have a drug-free, smoke-free policy in place for all employees, physicians, psychologists, therapists, and nurses?	——	——
2. Does the provider provide prompt, attentive service?	——	——
3. Does the provider endorse the World Class Quality Health Care philosophy?	——	——
4. Do diagnostic procedures include lifestyle, physical, and mental health assessments?	——	——
5. Is brief therapy available?	——	——
6. Is statistical process control used to constantly improve their quality of patient care services?	——	——
7. Are health education services available to meet your needs?	——	——
8. Is a prepared referral list of recommended self-help groups available?	——	——
9. Does the provider include the patient in physician, psychologist (or mental health therapist), and nurse team conferences?	——	——
10. Did the provider welcome your questions about their commitment to quality care?	——	——

A ready "Yes" answer to these questions suggests World Class Health Care. If your doctor is not familiar with the quality philosophy, share this book with him or her.

Unless our nation's families embrace World Class Health Care, the confrontational politics of Mothers Against Drunk Drivers (MADD) will serve as the political action model for our health care future.

Family Initiative

Families are our nation's most powerful political unit. Healthy families can give their members the support and encouragement which is needed to adopt the new health care philosophy. They can help each other establish and maintain good health habits. They can help every family member balance mental health and pursue lifelong health education.

Making a family decision to be healthy can be as arduous as pulling the plug on a terminal illness. Both decisions require consensus. Consensus is structured around common values and beliefs.

Beliefs and attitudes are a stronger bond than blood ties. Beliefs and attitudes must, therefore, be the focus of family negotiations. The preservation of health and the quality of a life to be led require negotiation. Negotiations may have to be limited to the immediate family or a circle of close friends. Negotiations are worthwhile because there is safety in numbers.

Opinions must be placed on the table. Awkward "if-the-time-comes" questions must be asked aloud. Promises to preserve health must be made sturdy. If they are weak a single decision by a father, mother, sister, or brother can entangle everyone in the unwinnable battle of bioethics.

Once a family envisions its picture of health, members must then decide how they will finance this identity. Health is an affordable option. If the family vision calls for heroic medical intervention, each member must know limited financial resources will one day ambush their plans. Hospital administrators and physicians can only support their vision until the money runs out. This has been and always will be the case.

Healthy family role models are abundant. They are worthy of study because clear behavior patterns emerge. Healthy families work for health. They have discovered good health is good fun. Good fun makes good health easier to practice. Practice develops skill. Skill leads to mastery. Health becomes a habit.

Unnecessary illness is avoided like the plague. The risks a family runs for heart disease, house fires, cancers, dental diseases, digestive disorders, respiratory diseases, infant mortality, and amputations related to vascular problems have been thrown out with the cigarettes.

Healthy families strive to meet the unique emotional needs of each family member. A respect for privacy is balanced with an understanding of the importance of family unity. Unity depends on time spent together. When family and friends cannot provide sufficient support, they employ trained counselors.

Healthy families know their family histories. Inherited diseases are given due consideration with assistance from qualified counselors of their choice. Any apparent genetic predisposition for alcoholism, drug addiction, domestic violence, child abuse, sexual abuse, depression, anxiety, psychosomatic disease, cancer, or cardiovascular disease is scrutinized using appropriate statistical process control tools. The risk for premature death and unnecessary illness need not be passed on from generation to generation.

A good partnership with a family physician is imperative. This long-term, intimate relationship builds an emotional bond that pays off handsomely in the physician's personal commitment to quality care. The physician's greatest gift is an ability to observe potential problems through personal interaction. Ask for, pay for, and encourage this type of service. Although physicians lack the counseling skill of a brief therapist and the polished style of an educator, conversations with your family doctor can be strong medicine.

Blood pressure checks, pap smears, prostate checks, and inoculations are helpful conversation bridges. Physicians skilled in the use of statistical thinking and control charts can use graphed data to search for patterns which suggest sexual problems, psychological distress, or the onset of a chronic disease which can handicap or end a life prematurely.

Good physicians are good teachers. They coax and coerce. They instruct. They role model good health habits and they look healthy. Good doctors refer to specialists in medicine, psychology, and education without hesitation because they respect their peers. The best doctors insist their patients have a comprehensive psychological assessment at least once every 10 years. The additional expense for these services is negligible. A health risk appraisal costs less than $10. A Minnesota Multiphasic Personality Inventory can be administered for under $20.

World Class Health Care doctors make sure their patients see a qualified nurse educator and mental health therapist during every office visit or hospital stay. Alcohol, drug, and depression inventories are taken every time. As we approach the twenty-first century, World Class Health Care physicians will make sure their patients understand and use the tools of statistical process control correctly.

Study the people and families you know who appear to be in good health. You are likely to find they are that way intentionally.

Employer Initiative

Health care costs equal and exceed the costs of raw materials for many manufacturing industries. They severely stress the service industries as well. High health care costs are deadlier than the disease W. Edwards Deming[5] diagnosed in his seminal work, *Out of the Crisis*. They are an issue of strategic importance to every business with an interest in survival. High health care costs are worthy of presidential attention.

Many people spend more time at work than they do with their families. Employers can use this reality to everyone's advantage. Time spent at work can and should contribute to employee health and well-being. The first return on investment employers will earn from this mind set is bigger profits.

Employers who make employee health a business priority will do seven things.

1. Adopt a World Class Health Care philosophy. Insist on the integration of medical science, behavioral science, education, and the use of statistical process control for all diagnosis and treatment interventions.
2. Build a consensus for quality.
3. Establish policies to screen job applicants for tobacco and drug use. Refuse to hire anyone who fails the screening.
4. Establish an off-site, confidential Employee Assistance Program or purchase an EAP service from a provider who can deliver evaluation, referral, and quality controlled brief therapy services.
5. Negotiate for quality, World Class Health Care service, and coverage. Expect an ever-increasing quality of service and ever-decreasing costs.
6. Establish a World Class Health Care supplier certification process.
7. Establish a costs of quality health care accounting system.

1. Adopt a World Class Health Care Philosophy

The president, chief executive officer, or owner of a business who adopts World Class Health Care must role-model good health habits. He or she must demonstrate a personal commitment to the World Class Health Care System. This leader must be a member of the team responsible for creating, purchasing, and administering World Class Health Care employee benefits and services.

The World Class Health Care philosophy empowers the team and other employees by creating the inspirational vision of a healthy, productive work force. Without this sense of future everyone remains stranded in the status quo. The best efforts at reducing health care costs will be futile.

2. Build a Consensus for Quality

High quality, low-cost health care is a new idea for anyone who has grown up believing in the "self-evident truth" that quality costs more, not less. World Class Health Care means as much change for buyers as it does for providers. Both have been victimized by obsolete thinking.

People need to buy into new ideas. Time is the coin of exchange in the idea marketplace.

Leaders who want to lead their organizations toward quality must spend time educating everyone. The more people know about how health care costs affect their jobs, salaries, families, and future in an international economy (fast becoming a global economy), the more willing they will be to help minimize those costs. The more people know about how to use World Class Health Care to their advantage, the more able they will be to take action.

Everyone in the organization must understand their link to the company's competitive position. When the work force views itself as a single population it will be able to focus its attention on changing its statistical shape (Figure 7.1).

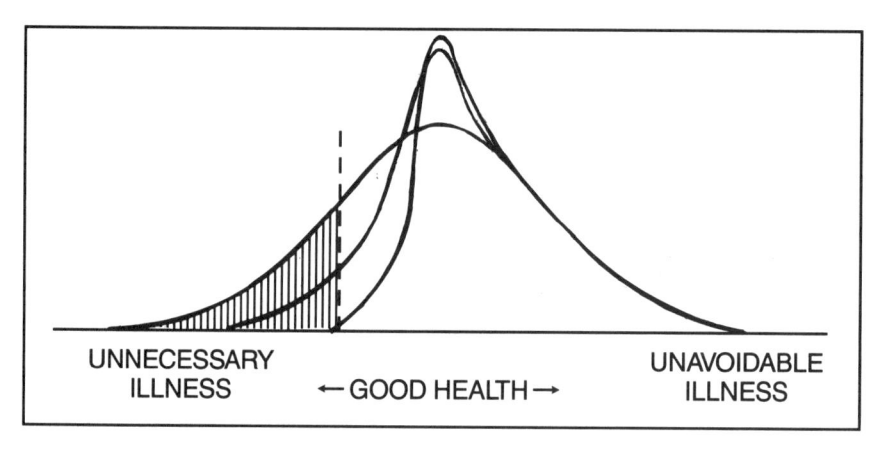

Figure 7.1 Health care expenses will be controlled when the population clusters nearer to the target (center) of the bell curve.

Health care expenses will come under control as the population clusters nearer to the target (center) of the bell curve. As these expenses are controlled the organization can choose to become more price competitive. A price competitive organization which delivers quality services and products stands an excellent chance for future growth and prosperity.

Prosperity is a political bandwagon people want to ride. The bandwagon will gain momentum each time an employee reaps a personal benefit from quality health care.

3. Establish an Employment Screening Policy

Once a person crosses over the line into alcohol and drug abuse and addiction, judgment, problem-solving ability, and integrity are compromised. Many abusers and almost all addicts have lost their ability to tell the truth. It is naive to think they can answer honestly when asked, "Do you abuse alcohol or drugs?"

Smokers still represent about 25 percent of our nation's population. Although their commitment to habit and nicotine may be strong, the lure of employment will give many a good reason to quit.

Since alcohol misuse, drug, and tobacco abuse are primary causes of high health care costs there is no reason to knowingly add this burden to the company cash flow. A simple pre-employment screening policy is a wise investment.

4. Establish an Employee Assistance Program

A confidential, company-wide Employee Assistance Program, an EAP, is an essential companion program to every pre-employment screening policy. Keeping humans healthy in the organization is as important as keeping high-risk employees out. The productivity losses and health insurance premium expenses caused by medical, surgical, and psychiatric service over-use, as well as mental health problems, alcohol and drug misuse and abuse, and tobacco use will hamper an organization's ability to compete in regional and local markets. A World Class Health Care EAP works to minimize these losses.

Chance life stressors place every human at risk for unhealthy behavior and destructive thinking. Financial problems, divorce, the loss of a loved one, and other special causes can and do disrupt the patterns of a healthy life. EAP counseling, referrals, and brief therapy can minimize the chaos and return an employee's lifestyle to a predictable state of statistical control.

The educational services which accompany good EAPs can change dietary and physical fitness habits as they transform the corporate culture. An EAP's brief psychotherapy service can keep the company's psychological health in balance as it builds a better bottom line.

5. Negotiate for Quality, World Class Health Care Service and Coverage

Outcome (Do my employees stay healthy?) and efficiency (Are my insurance premiums buying the best possible value at the lowest total cost?) are the best measures of health care quality. It is impossible to achieve either one without using statistical process control to integrate medical, mental health, and health education services. Both can be achieved by entering into a long-term partnership with a quality health care supplier willing to deliver World Class Health Care.

Quality patient care must be measured by the degree of process quality control and service integration a health care supplier achieves. A simple P chart can be used to monitor continuous decreases in bad outcomes. The number of hospitalizations or the percent defective, will be significantly reduced over time. Choosing a health care provider and a health care plan on their reputations for integrated services is sound thinking. Even when this precondition is met, astute negotiation will be required.

Negotiating teams must have a deep understanding of the political, economic, legislative, behavioral, and cultural obstacles which bar the path to World Class Health Care. Negotiators should have a working knowledge of hospital operations and insurance regulations. Each must be a strategist and a marketer.

World Class Health Care is an idea which will have to be sold to providers. Negotiators must be able to close the deal. An increasing number of first-rate medical centers, insurance companies, and mental health organizations are developing the capacity to deliver World Class Health Care. These are the health care suppliers which can hope to survive and flourish in the future.

Some hospitals have anticipated this opportunity. They are already using some World Class Health Care features to their advantage. They have nonsmoking senior level managers who represent medicine, behavioral science, nursing, education, and the marketing professions. They employ statisticians. They have pre-employment screening policies, well-run employee fitness programs, and easy to access EAP services in place.

These hospital managers possess sophisticated information systems. They understand the power of control charts and statistical reasoning. They have developed their ability to capitate medical, surgical, educational, and behavioral medicine services. Pressing these providers on price to secure the "cheapest" care dissuades them from applying their knowledge. A long-term commitment of market share will persuade them to use their skill.

6. Establish a Health Care Supplier Certification Process

A Health Care Supplier certification process which leads to a Basic Order Agreement can give employers the ability to establish the standards they want for employees: 100 percent World Class Health Care and 100 percent on-time delivery. See Appendix A for a sample certification program.

The general standards' categories every health care purchaser should review and negotiate with the health care supplier are outlined in a cause and effect diagram (Figure 7.2). A detailed breakdown of this diagram follows:

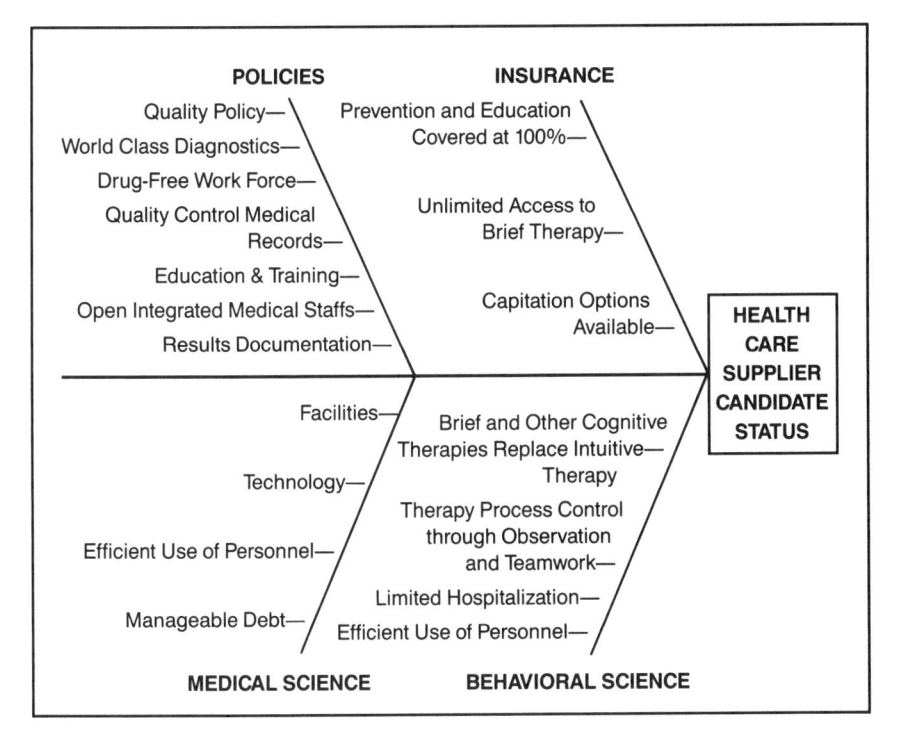

```
                    POLICIES              INSURANCE
            Quality Policy—      Prevention and Education
      World Class Diagnostics—      Covered at 100%—
       Drug-Free Work Force—
       Quality Control Medical        Unlimited Access to
                    Records—             Brief Therapy—
         Education & Training—
   Open Integrated Medical Staffs—    Capitation Options
                                          Available—          HEALTH
         Results Documentation—                                CARE
                                                              SUPPLIER
                   Facilities—                                CANDIDATE
                            Brief and Other Cognitive          STATUS
                          Therapies Replace Intuitive—
               Technology—            Therapy
                            Therapy Process Control
                               through Observation
      Efficient Use of Personnel—    and Teamwork—
                             Limited Hospitalization—
           Manageable Debt—  Efficient Use of Personnel—

               MEDICAL SCIENCE        BEHAVIORAL SCIENCE
```

Figure 7.2 Cause and effect diagram outlining general standards' categories to be negotiated with the health care supplier.

Policies

World Class Health Care treatment requires teamwork. All MDs, DOs, psychologists, mental health therapists, nurse educators, and patients are partners. The health care supplier's work force must share a commitment to the principles of the continuous improvement process articulated by Shewhart,[6] Deming,[5] Ishikawa,[7] Juran,[8] and others who champion the cause of continuous quality improvement. Their commitment will be evidenced by a meaningful corporate quality statement. We suggest the following:

> We are committed to the continuous improvement of health care services so the costs of care decrease forever. We share the savings we achieve with our customers through ever-decreasing prices.

Serious World Class Health Care providers will tie reputation to results. A primary quality benefit is lower costs. Lower costs can be shared with the customers.

World Class Health Care suppliers base every diagnosis on the results of disciplined data collection. Medical histories and physicals, lifestyle assessments, and behavioral medicine assessments are equally valued.

A World Class Health Care supplier willingly maintains a drug-free work force including all employees, physicians, nurses, therapists, and psychologists. World Class Health Care suppliers use statistical methods from the viewpoint of quality control. Data are always graphed over time. Medical records are written in a simple statistical language that all treatment team members can understand. All team members, including the patient, participate in quality of care process reviews.

Insurance

World Class Health Care insurers will offer quality indemnity insurance products aimed at reducing the costs of health care. They make insurance products available to the working poor who have made a commitment to healthy living. Their products will guarantee access to prevention. World Class Health Care insurance and health maintenance organization premiums must balance and reverse the incentives which promote health care service over use. Nonsmokers and nondrinkers who access prevention, education, and mental health services should enjoy low premiums. Smokers and drug abusers (alcohol is our culture's drug of choice) should pay high rates. Coverage benefits will no longer be based on the assumption that all customers want limitless life support technology. Benefits usually resemble the following model.

```
Hospitalization coverage ...................... 80–100%
Surgical services ................................ 80%
Medical services ................................. 80%
Mental health visits (limited) ..................... 50%
Alcohol and drug treatment (limited) ............... 50%
Minimal prevention service included free of charge.
```

Plans will no longer exclude mental health and alcohol/drug treatment services to "reduce" premium cost. Consequently, such problems as depression, alcohol misuse, and drug abuse will surface less frequently as medical and surgical problems.

World Class Health Care coverage will resemble the following model.

```
Prevention services, mental and physical health ...... 100%
Health education services ........................ 100%
World class diagnostics ........................... 90%
Outpatient and homecare medical services ........... 80%
Alcohol and drug treatment services ................ 80%
Outpatient surgery, medical and mental health care ... 60%
Inpatient surgery, medical and psychiatric care ....... 50%
Elective surgery ................................. 40%
```

Heroic end of life option packages ....
Multilevels of coverage available. Premiums based on current actuarial data, technology market prices, and number of customers in the heroic treatment risk pool.

World Class Health Care insurers will order World Class Health Care into use much in the same way health care purchasers order peer review of resource utilization today. Health care providers who fail to comply with World Class Health Care diagnostic and treatment protocols will not receive payment for services rendered. Those who fail to use statistical process control to continually improve their processes will be eliminated from the list of eligible health care suppliers.

Behavioral Medicine

Scientific, process focused, cognitive therapies will replace theoretical, psychoanalytic approaches to mental health care. Therapy quality and consistency will be controlled and replicated through teamwork and observation.

World Class Health Care suppliers possess the skill required to limit inpatient psychiatric hospitalizations to people who are a danger to themselves or others, people in need of protection, the chronically mentally ill, and patients with acute psychiatric disorders.

In the interest of cost-containment, psychiatrists are case medication monitors. Psychologists supervise the work of Master's level therapists.

Medical Science

The facilities, technologies, and personnel of medical science will remain as the most expensive health care components. Eric Trist[1], a founding member of the Tavistock Institute in London and a renowned systems theorist whose career spanned five decades, commented, "Hospitals are inherently sociotechnical as well as psychosocial, which accounts for the complexity of some of their dilemmas." The sociotechnical model Trist and others have developed is an ideal reference point for quality-minded health care organizations. A brief reading list on sociotechnical, systems thinking is provided at the end of this book.

Some of these expensive health care components are essential but World Class Health Care suppliers and customers will soon discover an important world class manufacturing lesson; world class quality is not a capital intensive process. Quality gains are largely made by maximizing the human element in every level of production process beginning with the supplier of raw materials.

Simplicity, flow-diagrammed jobs, job-specific training, an emphasis on superior housekeeping, constantly improved processes, just-in-time supply tactics, well-maintained equipment, quality circles, efficiently designed work units, and preventive maintenance, all minimize waste and needless complexity. Space, machines, and job functions once thought to be indispensable often can be eliminated.

Resilient good health, labor substitutions, and cross training minimize dependence on highly specialized workers. Teamwork and the principles of participation can replace technocratic bureaucracies.

Employers should review the capital debt obligations of potential World Class Health Care suppliers. A manageable debt will make a commitment to World Class Health Care possible.

7. Costs of Quality Health Care Accounting System

High health care costs rob profits from every employer in America. A simple costs of quality accounting system should be used to measure these losses. Juran,[8] the noted quality improvement thought leader, suggests the purpose of this management tool is to "illustrate the size of the quality problem and identify the projects for improvement."

"Costs of quality" is a phrase used to describe a useful management tool. A costs of quality accounting system measures two financial indicators: (1) investments made to produce quality, and (2) costs which result from using poor quality services and products.

A costs of quality accounting system is particularly appropriate for health care because investments made in World Class Health Care directly reduce total health care costs. Four elements must be included in the accounting system: prevention investment, appraisal investment, internal failure costs, and external failure costs.

Prevention Investments

These investments are incidental. The quality improvement literature is rich with examples of an average 10:1 return. When managed correctly they will rarely exceed $200 per employee or covered dependent per year. Investment categories include the following:

- Planning for quality care and quality control.
- Pre-employment drug screens.
- Drug, alcohol, and tobacco screens.
- Education expenses for teaching employees how to take advantage of World Class Health Care.

- Employee Assistance Program which includes unlimited access to brief therapy, stop smoking classes, and other health education opportunities.

Appraisal Investments

Quality improvement can be measured in dollars and cents. Computers, software, and existing accounting systems make the cost of tallying savings another incidental expense. The cost of a health care quality accounting and reporting system should function under the direction of the finance department.

Internal Failures

These costs can range from $2,500 to $5,000 per employee per year. Each company will have to determine its own cost. These costs include:

- Insurance premiums which result from alcohol and other drug abusers, smokers, and subscribers who avoid health education and defer mental health problems.
- Nonproductive time resulting from illness.
- Temporary help hired to cover absent employees.

External Failures

These costs are significant. Hospitalizations average $2,000 to $3,000 per day even for outpatient care. Bills for $50,000 to $100,000 are common. They include:

- Medical, surgical, and psychiatric inpatient hospitalizations.
- Suits against the company for unsafe working conditions.

Figure 7.3 shows one projection of a 10-year cost of quality health care report. Companies can expect to see better results through an aggressive application of the World Class Health Care philosophy.

The traditional costs of the quality model graphically summarizes the gains earned through quality improvement as shown in Figure 7.4. As quality investments increase, failure rates and the costs of quality are forced downward. When these two forces are combined on a single graph a zone of quality becomes visible. The goal is to move the zone toward 100 percent quality over time.

The quality zone target helps people visualize the forces of quality. Conceptual models are somewhat limited in what they can explain and

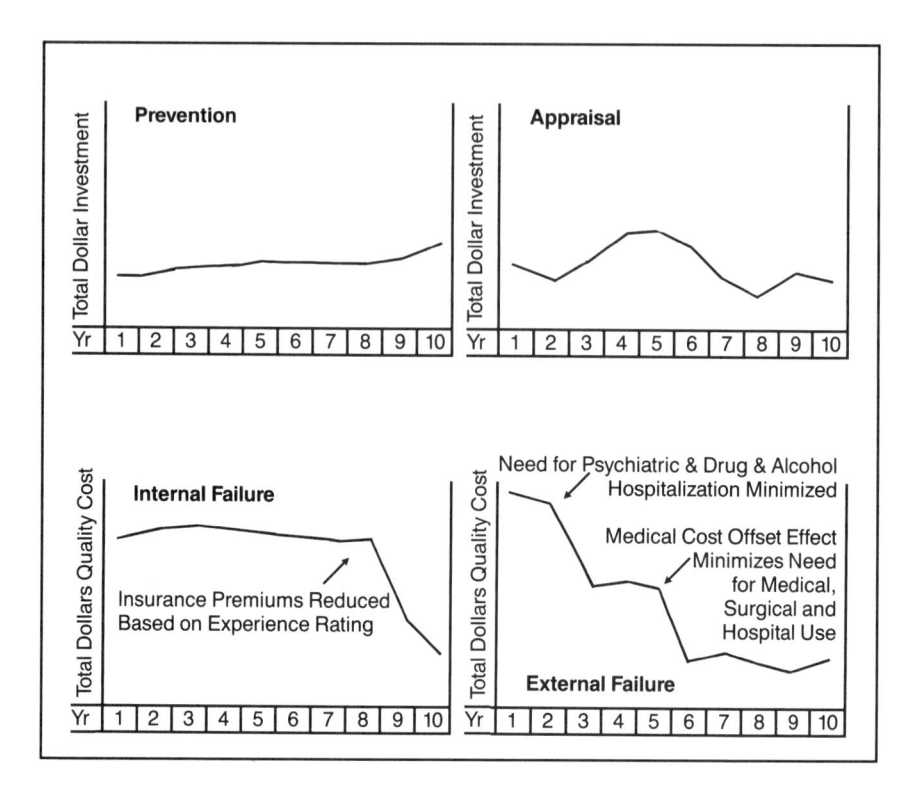

Figure 7.3 Projection of a ten year cost of quality health care report. *Adapted with permission from the American Society for Quality Control from H. James Harrington's* Poor Quality Costs, *page 90.*

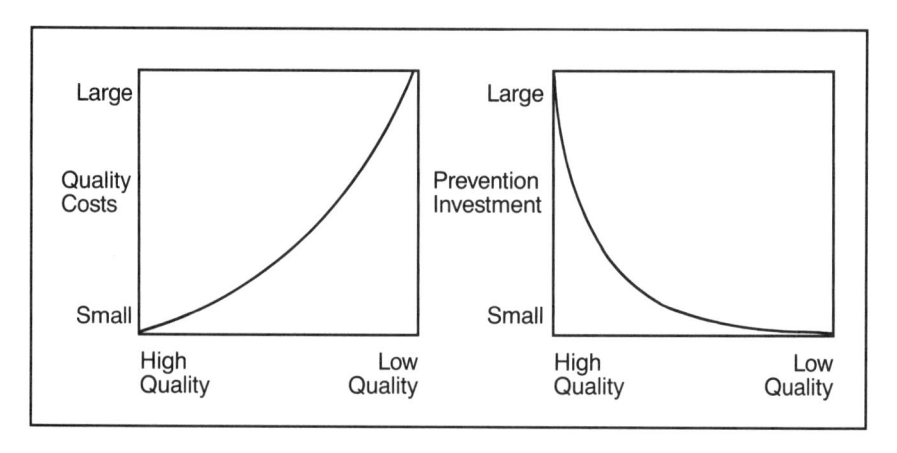

Figure 7.4 Traditional costs of quality model summarizing gains earned through quality improvement. *Adapted with permission from the American Society for Quality Control from H. James Harrington's* Poor Quality Costs, *pages 142 & 143.*

this one is no different. Theoretically, as quality nears 100 percent, prevention investments can be reduced. The valence of the groups of individuals that make up the total quality improvement cycle will hold quality gains in place.

The sooner an employer invests in a World Class Health Care partnership the sooner its health care costs will decrease (Figure 7.5). Decreasing health care costs will improve the employer's competitive position. A stronger competitive position will produce job security, more jobs, better wages, and bigger profits.

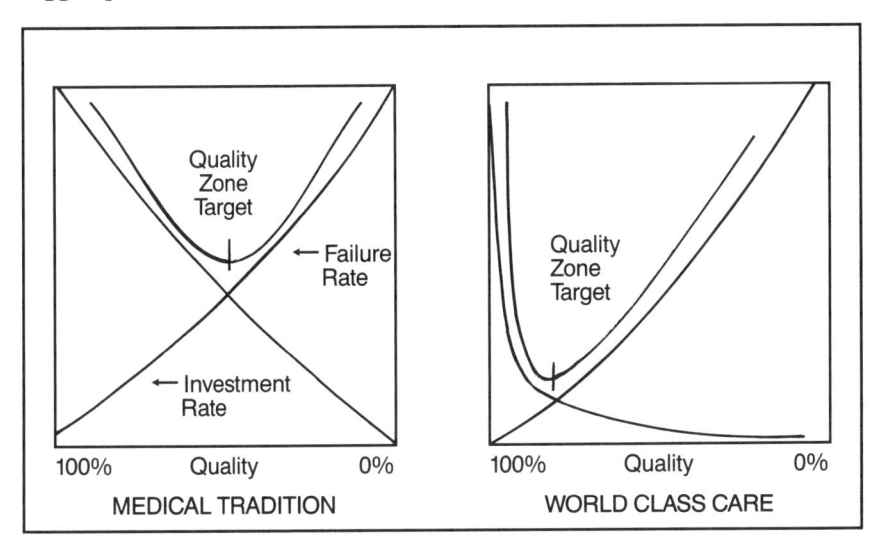

Figure 7.5 An increased investment in quality process improvement minimizes preventable illness. *Adapted with permission from the American Society for Quality Control from H. James Harrington's* Poor Quality Costs, *page 30.*

Congressional Initiative

Government has an obligation to serve and protect its citizens. Promoting the public health is a national defense issue. Our government buys such a large portion of our nation's health care output that it can choose to wield monopsony power in the public interest. Monopsony is the opposite of monopoly. Monopsony allows a single buyer to dictate prices.

Monopsony also gives the buyer an ability to demand World Class Health Care service. It can be used to forge a partnership with health care providers and insurers. These three partners—government, providers, and insurers—can design a World Class Health Care system. They can build quality into every health care treatment process. Their efforts will champion a decrease in total health care costs through continuous quality improvement; token proposals which call for increased spending to increase quality will be dismissed.

Since current national health care policies subsidize and reward inadequate diagnosis and inefficient treatment, congress will have to help us make some big changes. Congress must fund the development and design of a statistical, process-focused, World Class Health Care system. Shewhart[6] suggested five steps for developing a new manufacturing process. These five steps can be extremely useful to governmental, industrial, and health care service planning.

1. Study of the results of research to provide principles and numeric data on which to base a design.
2. Apply this information in the construction of a service delivery system designed to satisfy some human want, where no attention is given to cost.
3. Produce sample services under supposedly commercial conditions.
4. Test services for quality requirements, the reduction of illness, and health care expense.
5. Develop production methods.

Step 1 will be the most difficult step for our nation to take. Research results and the numeric data we use must be accurate. This book is not a statistical text. However, we assure readers the mistakes caused by inadequate data collection represent a minuscule piece of a colossal problem; none of our nation's health care data bases have been developed using the inductive reasoning of statistical method from the viewpoint of quality control.

The omission of vital mental health and lifestyle information by traditional diagnostics riddles our entire data base with error. The numbers our government uses for health care planning are further flawed by the deductive reasoning of mathematical statistics.

Mathematical statistics are not predictive. They are not capable of imparting predictive knowledge. A World Class Health Care system requires knowledge.

Good data must come from a controlled, constant system of chance causes. Constant errors of measurement and mistakes must be minimized or eliminated. Good data must provide a frame of reference for estimating the error of measurement. These requirements can be met when a process is brought into control using statistical methods from the viewpoint of quality control.

When a process, or a system of processes, is brought into control the continuous improvement process described by Deming[5] and Juran[8] can help us take Step 2. The public is crying out with their need for affordable, high-quality health care. We have an obligation to meet that market need especially since we have the knowledge and skill to meet the need economically.

Steps 3 and 4 can be made with knowledge we have today. Medical science, behavioral science, education, and statistical process control have proven and are proving their strength in the marketplace. The longer these disciplines stand alone in defense of their turf, the more expensive health care becomes. Together they are a powerful force for quality care and ever-diminishing health care costs.

Behavioral science has demonstrated the medical cost offset effect. Brief therapy can refine the existing model. A well-educated and therefore empowered public can learn to use all the health sciences efficiently.

Nurses contribute an enormous amount to our society. They can contribute more by working as full partners with physicians and psychologists.

The entire treatment team can enhance their productivity by working with safety engineers. Safety design has flexed its muscles and proven its value in the automotive industry. Injury-proofed cars are only a first step. Injury-proofed work stations must become a priority for employers and employees alike.

The statistically controlled quality production methods required by Step 5 have existed for more than 60 years. They are evidenced by KAIZEN[9] in Japan. They work for scores of World Class Manufacturing companies from France, Holland, and the United States of America. Such companies as Xerox, IBM, Ford, AT&T, Kodak, Hewlett-Packard, Florida Power and Light, Motorola, GM, Weyerhauser, Milliken, and hundreds of others know the quality improvement process produces delighted customers. Continuous quality improvement permits competitive pricing. It creates a long-term competitive advantage for the quality company.

Thomas Kuhn[10] described the structure of scientific revolutions. Shewhart[6] provided theory. When we know the theory we can control the revolution of World Class Health Care.

Congress need only fund the cause of teamwork between four proven disciplines: medical science, behavioral science, education, and statistical method from the viewpoint of quality control.

Comment

Someday soon patients will be given the power to participate fully in their care. Prevention, education, behavioral science, and statistical process control will lighten the unsafe load we have placed on traditional technologies.

A World Class Health Care value payment system will soon replace the perverse incentives of the old *Relative Value System*. Education and prevention will have priority by the year 2010. In the meantime, those of us who are dedicated to World Class Health Care shall continue to try to heal and treat people after they have gotten themselves into trouble.

Many of us will work to create a World Class Health Care delivery system where medical science, behavioral science, health education, and process quality control work together for optimal patient outcomes. More money will be tossed into the wishing well of literature by people who believe words can change people. Other books will be written and new organizations will be formed.

Finally, a day will come when we are guaranteed access to World Class Health Care. We will take care of ourselves with an integrated, cooperative support network of medical doctors, behavioral science physicians, and skilled nurse educators.

Envision a future where the quality of preventive health care is so high that today's health care system is remembered as needless complexity. Envision a future where health care industry professionals possess profound knowledge; the higher the quality of health services delivered, the lower the total costs of care will be. Lower total costs improve access to health care services for all citizens.

REFERENCES

1. Trist, E. *The Evolution of Socio-Technical Systems.* A conceptual framework and action research program, occasional paper no. 2. Ontario Ministry of Labour, Ontario Quality of Working Life Center, June 1981.

2. Starr, P. *The Social Transformation of American Medicine, the Rise of a Sovereign Industry.* New York: Basic Books, 1982.

3. Hamilton, E. M., and E. Whitney. *Nutrition Concepts and Controversies.* St. Paul, MN: West Publishing.

4. Cooper, K. O. *Aerobics.* New York: Bantam, 1968.

5. Deming, E. *Out of the Crisis.* Cambridge: Massachusetts Institute of Technology, 1988.

6. Shewhart, W. A. *Economic Control of Quality of Manufactured Product.* New York: Macmillan and Van Nostrand, 1931. Commemorative reissue Milwaukee: ASQC Quality Press, 1980.

7. Ishikawa, K. "What Is Total Quality Control?" In *Quality Control Handbook,* edited by K. Ishikawa. Englewood Cliffs, NJ: Prentice-Hall, 1985.

8. Juran, J. M. *Juran's Quality Control Handbook.* 4th ed. New York: McGraw-Hill, 1988.

9. Masaaki, I. *Kaizen.* New York: Random House, 1986.

10. Kuhn, T. S. *The Structure of Scientific Revolution.* Chicago: University of Chicago Press, 1970.

EPILOGUE 2010

David Solomon is president of County College Health Sciences Center. His wife Sarah quit her catering business and returned to nursing. She is the executive director of City College's Education and Referral Division.

Roy and Helen just celebrated their 52nd wedding anniversary. Roy's defibrillator works just fine.

Matthew Jobe manages Colorado's Emergency Medicine Services Network and the Western Region Rural Prevention Services Network. His ambulances hardly ever leave their garages but he is glad there are enough people and equipment to respond should the need arise.

Mrs. Jameson and Tommy moved to Hawaii in 1990. They both love to surf.

Mr. Pitstick has been clean and sober since 1990. None of his children drink. Joanie claims they have never been happier.

Mr. and Mrs. Richards were sentenced to six months probation. They died in a high-speed automobile accident two days after sentencing. Neither one was wearing a seat belt. Both had been drinking.

Mr. Taylor lived in the Intensive Care Unit of County Hospital for six months. He was finally allowed to die after his wife divorced him and declared bankruptcy. Mr. Taylor's bill totaled $360,000.

Perry drives the ER rig for County College Health Sciences Center. He thinks teaching is the best part of his job.

Mr. Martin died in 1994 of a cold.

Mr. and Mrs. Hahn retired on their $50 million jackpot from the Colorado State Lottery in 1992. They donated $500,000 to County Hospital as a trust fund to educate low-income expectant parents. Some of the money has been used for a film library.

Tim is the vice president of marketing for County College Health Sciences Center. He buys more than $4 million in advertising each year. Business is booming. The customers are delighted.

John is teaching brief therapy and service integration theory at Harvard.

Bertha retired in 1998 to care for her grandchildren, or "little duckies," as she prefers to call them.

Dr. Bob became unemployed when technology rendered heart surgery obsolete in 1999. He made a killing in real estate and hasn't worked at all since 2001.

Larry is a certified brief therapist. He practices his profession in Seattle, Washington.

Kyle overdosed on cocaine at age 14.

SOURCES AND RECOMMENDED READING

Fuchs, V. R. *Who Shall Live? Health, Economics and Social Change.* New York: Basic Books, 1974.

HEALTH CARE CHAOS

(Note: *The Surgeon General's Report on Healthy People* and *The Carter Center Study* are documents of historical proportion. The facts we cited came from their data analysis.

Specific readings of interest are:

Amler, R. W., and H. B. Dull. *Closing the Gap.* New York: Oxford Press, 1987.

Armstrong, B., and R. Doll. "Environmental Factors in Cancer Incidents in Mortality in Different Countries with Special Reference to Dietary Practices." *International Journal of Cancer* 15 (1975): 617-631.

Bayer, R. "The Care of the Terminally Ill: Mortality and Economics." *New England Journal of Medicine* (December 15, 1983): 1490-1494.

Bloom, B. S., and P. D. Kissick. "Home and Hospital Costs of Terminal Illness." *Medical Care* 18, No. 5 (May 1980): 560-564.

Berkelman, R. L., et al. "Fatal Injuries in Alcohol." *American Journal of Preventative Medicine* (1985): 1:21-28.

Brodaty, H., G. Andrews, and L. Kehoe. "Psychiatric Illness in General Practice I; Why Is it Missed?" *Australian Family Physician* 11, No. 8: (August 1982): 625-631.

Bronstein, J. M., and C. A. Jones. "Ethics, Technology and the High Cost of Dying: A Public Forum." *Southern Medicine Journal* 79, No. 12 (December 1986): 1485-1488.

Collins, J. *Drinking in Crime.* New York: Guilford, 1981.

Christopherson, B., and C. Pieffer. "Varying the Timing of Information to Alter Preoperative Anxiety and Postoperative Recovery in Cardiac Surgery Patients." *Heart and Lung* 9, No. 5 (1980): 854-861.

Civetta, J. M. "The Inverse Relationship Between Cost and Survival." *Journal of Surgical Research* 14 (1973): 265-269.

Deming, E. *Out of the Crisis.* Cambridge: Massachusettes Institute of Technology, 1988.

Derlet, R. W. "Emergency Department Presentation of Cocaine Intoxication." *Annals of Emergency Medicine* 18, No. 2 (February 1989): 182-186, 115-119.

Devine, E. C., and T. D. Cook. "The Meta-analytic Analysis of Effects of Psychoeducational Interventions on Length of Postsurgical Hospital Stay." *Nursing Research* 32, No. 5 (September/October 1985): 267-274.

Duhl, L. J., N. A. Cummings, and J. J. Hynes. "The Emergence of the Mental Health Complex." *Psychiatry Annals* 16, No. 8 (August 1986): 442-447.

Feldman, L., and V. Goldman. "Mental Health Care in HMOs: Practice and Potential." *Psychiatry Annals* 16, No. 8 (August 1986): 463-469.

Fell, J. C. "Alcohol Involvement in Traffic Accidents: Recent Estimates from the National Center for Statistics in Analysis." Washington, DC: Department of Transportation, 1982; Report No. DOT HS-806 269.

Ford, G. R., and J. Carter. *American Agenda, Report to the Forty-First President of the United States of America,* 1988.

Gelles, R. J. *The Violent Home.* Beverly Hills, CA: Sage Publications, 1974.

Gordon, E., et al. "A Neurophysiological Study of Somatization Disorder." *Comprehensive Psychiatry* 27, No. 4 (July/August 1986): 295-301.

Kassakian, M. G., et al. "The Cost and Quality of Dying: A Comparison of Home and Hospital." *Nurse Practitioner* (Jan/Feb 1979): 18-23.

Lloyd, G. G. "Review Article Psychiatric Syndromes with a Somatic Presentation." *Journal of Psychosomatic Research* 30, No. 2 (1986): 113-20.

Lowering Blood Cholesterol to Prevent Heart Disease: Consensus Development Conference Statement. National Institutes of Health, Bethesda, MD, Small Bol. 5, No. 7. 1985.

Long, S. "Medical Expenditures of Terminal Cancer Patients During the Last Year of Life." *Inquiry* 21 (Winter 1984): 315-327.

Miller, G. 1987. House of Representatives, California. Congressional record—extensions of remarks. Wed. Sept. 23.

McCall, N. "Utilization and Costs of Medicare Services by Beneficiaries in the Last Year of Life." *Medical Care* 22, No. 4 (1984):329-342.

Miller, N. S., M. S. Gold, and R. L. Millman. "Cocaine." *American Family Physician* 39, No. 2 (February 1989):115-120.

Moore, R. D., et al. "Prevalence, Detection and Treatment of Alcoholism in Hospitalized Patients." *JAMA* 261, No. 3 (January 1989): 403-407.

Pollack, E. S., et al. "Perspective Study of Alcohol Consumption in Cancer." *New England Journal of Medicine* 310 (1984): 617-621.

Quill, T. E. "Somatization Disorder: One of Medicine's Blind Spots." *JAMA* 254, No. 21 (December 1985): 3075-3079.

Regier, D. A., et al. "The NIMH Depression Awareness, Recognition, and Treatment Program: Structure, Aims, and Scientific Basis." *American Journal of Psychiatry* 145, No. 11 (November 1989): 1351-1357.

Scitovsky, A. A. "The High Cost of Dying: What Do the Data Show?" *Health and Society* 62, No. 4 (1984): 591-608.

Southgate, M. T. "Hypochondriasis and Somatization." *JAMA* 258, No. 19 (1987): 2718-2722.

Stoudemire, A. "Depression in the Medically Ill." In *Psychiatry*, Vol. 2, edited by J. O. Cavenar. New York: Lippincott, 1985.

Stewart, S., et al. "Functional Status and Well-being of Patients with Chronic Conditions." *JAMA* 262, No. 7 (August 1989): 907-913.

Surgeon General. *Healthy people: Surgeon General's Report on Health Promotion and Disease Prevention.* Washington, DC: GPO, 1979.

Swartz, M., et al. "Somatization Disorder in a Community Population." *American Journal of Psychiatry* 143, No. 11 (November 1986): 1403-1408.

Swartz, M., D. Hughes, and D. Blazer, et al. "Somatization Disorder in the Community a Study of Diagnostic Concordance Among Three Diagnostic Systems." *Journal of Nervous and Mental Diseases* 175, No. 1 (1987): 26-33.

Wells, H. G., B. Kenneth, and A. Stewart, et al. "The Functioning and Well-being of Depressed Patients." *JAMA* 262, No. 7 (August 1989): 914-919.

Wechsler, H. "Alcohol Level and Home Accidents." *Public Health Reports* 84 (1969): 1043-1969.

Wolfgang, M. E. *Patterns of Criminal Homicide.* New York: Wiley, 1958.

Zahn, M. A. "Drug Use in the Structure of Homicide in Two US Cities." *In the New and Old Criminology*, edited by E.E. Flynn and J.P. Comrade. New York: Prager, 1978.

MEDICAL COST OFFSET EFFECT

Cummings, N. A., and W. R. Follette. "Psychiatric Services and Medical Utilization in a Prepaid Health Plan Setting: Part II." *Medical Care* 6, No. 1 (January-February 1968): 31-41.

Cummings, N. A. "Prolonged (Ideal) Versus Short-Term (Realistic) Psychotherapy." *Professional Psychology* (November 1977): 491-501.

Cummings, N. A., and L. J. Duhl. "The New Delivery System." *Psychiatric Annals* 16, No. 8 (August 1986): 470-475.

Follette, W. T., and N. A. Cummings. "Psychiatric Services and Medical Utilization in a Prepaid Health Plan Setting: Part I." *Medical Care* 5, No. 1 (January-February 1967): 25-35.

Goldberg, I. D., G. Krantz, and B. Z. Locke. "Effects of Short-term Outpatient Psychiatric Therapy Benefit on the Utilization of Medical Services in a Prepaid Group Practice Medical Program." *Medical Care* 8, No. 5 (September/October 1970): 419-428.

Goldensohn, S. S., and R. Fink. "Mental Health Services for Medicaid Enrollees in a Prepaid Group Practice Plan." *American Journal of Psychiatry* 136, No. 2 (February 1979): 160-164.

Holder, H. D., and J. O. Blose. "Changes in Healthcare Costs and Utilization Associated with Mental Health Treatment." *Hospital and Community Psychiatry* 38, No. 10 (October 1987): 1070-1075.

Lehman, A. F. "Capitation Payment and Mental Health Care: A Review of the Opportunities and Risks." *Hospital and Community Psychiatry* 38, No. 1 (January 1987): 31-38.

Mumford, E., H. J. Schlesinger, and G. V. Glass. "The Effects of Psychological Intervention on Recovery from Surgery and Heart Attacks: and Analysis of the Literature." *American Journal of Preventive Health* 72, No. 2 (February 1982): 141-151.

Mumford, E., et al. "A New Look at Evidence About Reduced Cost of Medical Utilization Following Mental Health Treatment." *American Journal of Psychiatry* 141, No. 10 (October 1984): 1145-1158.

Sperling, M. *Psychosomatic Disorders in Childhood.* New York: Jason Aronson, 1978.

Shemo, J. P. D. "Cost-effectiveness in Medicine of Providing Mental Health Services: The Offset Effect." *International Journal of Psychiatry* 15, No. 1 (1985-1986): 19-29.

White, S. L. "The Impact of Mental Health Services on Medical Care Utilization: Economic and Organizational Implications." *Hospital Community Psychiatry* 32, No. 5 (May 1981): 311-19.

BRIEF THERAPY

Broadaty, H., and G. Andrews. "Brief Psychotherapy in Family Practice: A Controlled Prospective Intervention Trial." *British Journal of Psychiatry* 143, No. 11 (1983): 11-19.

deShazer, H., and I. K. Berg, et al. "Brief Therapy: Focused Solution Development." *Family Process* 25 (June 1986): 207-221.

deShazer, L. *Keys to Solution in Brief Therapy.* New York: W.W. Norton and Company.

deShazer, S. *Clues—Investigating Solutions in Brief Therapy.* New York: W.W. Norton and Company, 1988.

deShazer, S. "A Requiem for Power." *Contemporary Family Therapy* (Summer 1988): 69-76.

Fisch, R., J. H. Weakland, and L. Segal. *The Tactics of Change, Doing Therapy Briefly.* San Francisco: Jossey Bass Publishers, 1982.

Gillet, R. "Short-Term Intensive Psychotherapy: A Case History." *British Journal of Psychiatry* 148 (1986): 98-100.

Kaskey, G. "Brief Psychiatric Inpatient Care for Acutely Disturbed Patients." *Hospital Community Psychiatry* 38, No. 11 (November 1987): 1203-1206.

Logsdon, D. N. and M. A. Rosen. "The Cost of Preventative Health Services in Primary Medical Care and Implications for Health Insurance Coverage." *Journal of Ambulatory Care Management* 7 (November 1984): 46-55.

Logsdon, D. N., et al. "Coverage of Preventive Services by Preferred Provider Organizations." *Journal of Ambulatory Care Management* 10 (May 1987): 25-35.

Molnar, A., and S. deShazer. "Solution-Focused Therapy: Toward the Identification of Therapeutic Tasks." *Journal of Marital Family Therapy* 13, No. 4 (1987): 349-58.

Weiner-Davis, M., S. deShazer, and W. J. Gingerich "Building on Pretreatment Change to Construct the Therapeutic Solution: An Exploratory Study." *Journal of Marital Family Therapy* 13, No. 4 (1987): 359-363.

Zweven, A., and S. Pearlman. "Evaluating the Effectiveness of Conjoint Treatment of Alcohol Complicated Marriages: Clinical and Methodological Issues." *Journal of Marital Family Therapy* 9 (1983): 61-72.

Zweben, A., S. Pearlman, and S. Li. "A Comparison of Brief Advice and Conjoint Therapy in the Treatment of Alcohol Abuse: The Results of the Marital Systems Study." *British Journal of Addiction* 83 (1988): 899-916.

EDUCATION AND SELF-HELP

For information on three-hour, lifestyle change programs *Positive Pulse, A Program to Promote Healthy Lifestyles* and *Backup, A Program to Prevent Back Pain* contact United General Hospital in Sedro-Woolley, Washington.

The American Cancer Society, the American Heart Association, the American Lung Association, Planned Parenthood, the Dairy Council, Alcoholics Anonymous, the National Self-Help Clearinghouse, and scores of other organizations have outstanding educational programs and materials.

Gintner, G. G. "Relapse Prevention in Health Promotion: Strategies and Long-term Outcome." *Journal of Mental Health Counseling* 10, No. 2 (1988): 123-135.

Maton, K. I. "Social Support, Organizational Characteristics, Psychological Well-Being, and Group Appraisals in Three Self-Help Group Populations." *American Journal of Community Psychology* 16, No. 1 (1988): 53-77.

Weinstein, N. D. "Effects of personal Experience on Self-protective Behavior." *Psychology Bulletin* 105, No. 1 (1989): 31-50.

Woolert, R. W., L. H. Levy, and B. G. Knight. "Help Giving in Behavioral Control and Stress Coping Self-help Groups." *Small Group Behavior* 13, No. 2 (May 1982): 204-218.

WORLD CLASS HEALTH CARE

Beck, A. T. *Depression: Causes and Treatment.* Philadelphia: University of Pennsylvania Press, 1972.

Beck, A. T., R. A. Steer, and M. G. Garbin. "Psychometric Properties of the Beck Depression Inventory: Twenty-Five Years of Evaluation." *Clinical Psychology Review* 8 (1988): 77-100.

Cleary, P. D., et al. "Prevalence and Recognition of Alcohol Abuse in a Primary Care Population." *American Journal of Medicine* 85 (October 1988): 466-471.

Cyr, M. G., and S. A. Wartman. "The Effectiveness of Routine Screening Questions in the Detection of Alcoholism." *JAMA* 259, No. 1 (January 1988): 51-54.

Deming, W. E. *Out of the Crisis.* Cambridge: Massachusetts Institute of Technology, 1988.

Einstein, A. *Relativity.* New York: Crown Books, 1959.

Garvin, D. A. *Managing Quality.* New York: Free Press, 1987.

Gitlow, H., and S. Gitlow. *The Deming Guide to Quality and Competitive Position.* Englewood Cliffs, NJ: Prentice Hall, 1986.

Feigenbaum, A. V. *Total Quality Control.* New York: McGraw Hill, 1983.

Harrington, H. J. *Poor Quality Costs.* Milwaukee: ASQC Quality Press, 1987.

Imai, M. *Kaizen.* New York: Random House, 1986.

Ishikawa, K. What is Total Quality Control? In *Quality Control Handbook,* edited by K. Ishikawa. Englewood Cliffs, NJ: Prentice Hall, 1985.

Juran, J. M. *Juran on Planning for Quality.* New York: Free Press, 1988.

Juran, J. M. *Managerial Breakthrough.* New York: McGraw Hill, 1964.

Juran, J. M. *Juran's Quality Control Handbook.* 4th ed. New York: McGraw Hill, 1988.

Kuhn, T. S. *The Structure of Scientific Revolution.* Chicago: University of Chicago Press, 1962.

Lewis, C. I. *Mind and the World Order, Outline of a Theory of Knowledge.* New York: Dover Press, 1929.

Ott, E. O. *Process Quality Control: Troubleshooting and Interpretation of Data.* New York: McGraw-Hill, 1975.

Rosander, A. C. *Applications of Quality Control in the Service Industries.* Milwaukee: ASQC Quality Press, 1985.

Scherkenbach, W. W. *The Deming Route to Quality and Productivity: Road Maps and Roadblocks.* Washington, DC: CEEP Press, 1988.

Scholtes, P. *The Team Handbook.* Madison, WI: Joiner and Associates, 1988.

Selzer, M. L. "The Michigan Alcoholism Screening Test: The Quest for a New Diagnostic Instrument." *American Journal of Psychiatry* 12 (June 1971): 89-94.

Shewhart, W. A. *Economic Control of Quality of Manufactured Product.* New York: Macmillan and Van Norstrand, 1931. Commemorative reissue Milwaukee: ASQC Quality Press, 1980.

Shewhart, W. A. *Statistical Method from the Viewpoint of Quality Control.* New York: Dover Publications, 1939.

STATISTICAL PROCESS CONTROL

Box, G., W. Hunter, and J. Hunter. *Statistics for Experimenters.* New York: John Wiley and Sons, 1978.

Duncan, A. J. *Quality Control and Industrial Statistics.* Homewood, IL: Business One Irwin, 1986.

Hicks, C. R. *Fundamental Concepts in Design of Experiments.* New York: Holt, Rinehart and Winston, 1982.

Neter, J., W. Wasserman, and M. Kutner. *Applied Linear Statistical Models.* Homewood, IL: Business One Irwin, 1985.

SOCIO-TECHNICAL ORGANIZATIONAL DESIGN

Emery, F. E. "Characteristics of Socio-Technical Systems." London: Tavistock Documents #527. Abridged in F.E. Emery, *The Emergence of a New Paradigm of Work.* Canberra: Centre for Continuing Education.

Trist, E. *The Evolution of Socio-Technical Systems, a conceptual framework and action research program,* occasional paper no. 2. Ontario Ministry of Labour, Ontario Quality of Working Life Centre, June 1981.

von Bertalanffy, L. "The Theory of Open Systems in Physics and Biology." *Science* 3 (1950): 23-29.

von Bertalanffy, L. *General System Theory.* New York: George Braziller, 1968.

GENERAL READING

Armor, D. J. "The RAND Reports and the Analysis of Relapse." In *Alcoholism: New Knowledge and New Responses,* edited by G. Edwards and M. Grant. Baltimore: University Park Press, 1976.

Amler, R. W., and H. B. Dull. "Closing the Gap: The Burden of Unnecessary Illness." *American Journal of Preventive Medicine* 3, No. 5 (1987).

Carels, E. J. "The Cost-Effectiveness of Alcoholism Treatment." *The CareMedic* (May 1979): 2-6.

Frazier, S. H., and D. L. Parron "The Federal Mental Health Agenda." *Psychiatry Annals* 16, No. 8 (August 1986): 448-458.

Fingerette, H. *Heavy Drinking: The Myth of Alcoholism as a Disease.* Berkeley, CA: University of California Press, 1988.

Griffin, G. C. "What I Didn't Know Almost Killed Me." *Postgrad Medicine* 84, No. 3 (1988): 13-14.

Hayami, D. E., and D. K. Freborn. "Effect of Coverage on Use of an HMO Alcoholism Treatment Program: Outcome and Medical Care Utilization." *AJPH* 71, No. 10 (1981): 1133-1143.

Hegyvary, S. T., and P. A. Chamings. "The Hospital Setting and Patient Care Outcomes." *Journal of Nursing Administration* 5, No. 3 (March/April 1975): 29-32.

Hilgard, E. R., and G. H. Bower. *Theories of Learning*, 3rd ed. Century Psychology Series. New York: Appleton Century Crofts, 1966.

Jameson, J., L. J. Shuman, and W. W. Young. "The Effects of Outpatient Psychiatric Utilization on the Costs of Providing Third-party Coverage." *Medical Care* 16, No. 5 (May 1987): 383-399.

Karasu, T. B. "The Psychotherapies: Benefits and Limitations." *American Journal of Psychotherapy* 40, No. 3 (July 1986): 324-343.

Kogan, W. S., et al. "Impact of Integration of Mental Health Service and Comprehensive Medical Care." *Medical Care* 13, No. 1 (November 1975): 934-942.

Koss, M. P., J. N. Butcher, and H. H. Strupp. "Brief Psychotherapy Methods in Clinical Research." *Journal of Consulting and Clinical Psychology* 54, No. 1 (1986): 60-67.

Levinson, H. "What Killed Bob Lyons?" *Harvard Business Review* (March/April, 1981): 144-162.

Levitan, S. J., and D. S. Kornfeld. "Clinical and Cost Benefits of Liaison Psychiatry." *American Journal of Psychiatry* 138, No. 6 (June, 1981): 790-793.

McHugh, J. P., M. W. Kahn, and E. Heiman. "Relationships Between Mental Health Treatment and Medical Utilization Among Low-income Mexican-American Patients: Some Preliminary Findings." *Medical Care* 5, No. 5 (May 1977): 439-444.

Masters, J. C., and R. Spilter. "Neuroleptic Malignant Syndrome." *Journal of Psychosocial Nursing* 24, No. 9 (September 1986): 11-16.

Morrow, P. L., J. G. Thompson, and J. M. Cunningham. "To Bedlam and Back." *Journal of Psychosocial Nursing* 24, No. 9 (September 1986): 17-20.

Norfleet, M. A., and G. M. Burnell. "Utilization of Medical Services by Psychiatric Patients." *Hospital Community Psychiatry* 32, No. 3 (March 1981): 198-200.

Pincus, H. A. "Making the Case for Consultation-liaison Psychiatry: Issues in Cost-effectiveness Analysis." *General Hospital Psychiatry* 6 (1984): 173-179.

Rinsley, D. B. "Successful Treatment of a Case of Ocular Tic Utilizing Brief, Intensive Psychoanalytic Psychotherapy." *Bull Menninger Clinic* 50, No. 5 (1986): 447-455.

Robinson, M. L. "HHS Considers Medicare MD Franchises." *Hospitals* (November 1987): 28-29.

Rosen, J. C., and A. N. Wiens. "Changes in Medical Problems and Use of Medical Services Following Psychological Intervention." *American Psychology* 34, No. 5 (May 1979): 420-431.

Schlesinger, H. J., E. Mumford, and G. V. Glass. "Mental Health Treatment and Medical Care Utilization and a Fee-for-Service System: Outpatient Mental Health Treatment Following the Onset of Chronic Disease." *American Journal of Preventive Health* 73, No. 4 (April 1983): 422-429.

Scheffler, R. M. "The Economics of Mental Health Care." *Psychiatry Annals* 16, No. 8 (August 1986): 460-462.

Smith, G. R., L. M. Miller, and R. A. Monson. "Consultation-Liaison Intervention in Somatization Disorder." *Hospital Community Psychiatry* 37, No. 12 (December 1986): 1207-1210.

Thomas, M. D., E. Sanger, and J. D. Whitner. "Nursing Diagnosis of Depression." *Journal of Psychosocial Nursing* 24, No. 8 (August 1986): 6-12.

Wallace, C. "Employers Turning to Managed Care to Control Their Psychiatric Care Costs." *Modern Healthcare* 17, No. 14 (July 1987): 82-84.

Weissberg, J. H. "Short-Term Dynamic Psychotherapy: An Application of Psychoanalytic Personality Theory." *Journal of the American Academy of Psychoanalysis* 12, No. 1 (1984): 101-113.

Weissberg, J. H. "The Therapeutic Relationship in Brief Focal Psychotherapy." *Journal of the American Academy of Psychoanalysis* 14, No. 2 (1986): 203-212.

Zoccolillo, M. and C. R. Cloninger. "Somatization Disorder: Psychologic Symptoms, Social Disability, and Diagnosis." *Comprehensive Psychiatry* 27, (January/February 1986): 65-73.

APPENDIX A

Sample Certification Program

Supplier certification programs are commonplace among quality manufacturers. The mutual dedication of supplier and producer to the quality philosophy creates benefits for the customer.

The StorageTek Process Quality Rating Program is a good model. Hospitals, physicians, behavior medicine professionals, and other health care providers who adapt a framework similar to this program will be able to accelerate their quality improvement programs. The higher the quality the lower the cost.

Acknowledgment is given to Storage Technology Corporation and Mr. George Eckes, manager of the Supplier Quality Assistance Group for permission to use the Process Quality Rating (PQR) document. This document was conceived and developed by the Supplier Quality Assistance Group to obtain an objective evaluation of a supplier's individual process improvement system and associated activities. The evaluation of this document and the subsequent mutual action plan helps to drive ongoing process improvement through the StorageTek supplier base.

PROCESS QUALITY RATING (PQR)

INTRODUCTION

Today, Quality Improvement is emphasized as a necessary element to sustain and increase market share. Unfortunately, misconceptions abound with regard to what Quality Improvement is and how to achieve it. StorageTek's Process Quality Rating (PQR) will assist you, the Supplier, in determining the extent and effectiveness of your Quality Improvement efforts.

The PQR is a comprehensive tool that shows Quality Improvement as more than data collection, control charting, or a quality circle. It will allow you to gauge your overall performance with regard to Quality Improvement. More importantly, it will show where you can focus your efforts to achieve the goal of lower production costs through better quality. This, of course, can only lead to more customer exposure and ultimately larger market share. In this manner, you can become not only a better Supplier to StorageTek, but a leader in your respective industry.

Therefore, the ultimate purpose is to use the PQR as a vehicle to assist in making your Quality Improvement efforts more efficient and cost effective. While a numerical ranking is generated, less attention should be placed on that number and more attention should be placed on those areas that need improvement.

Along with the completed PQR, verification of each element is required to allow an objective evaluation. Please note the verification requirements listed at the end of each section of the PQR. **Without this verification, no credit is given.** This verification must be current and be on file at StorageTek or accompany the completed PQR.

As always, StorageTek's Quality Assistance Group is available to assist you with efforts at making your program more efficient and productive.

APPENDIX A

COMPANY _____

COMPLETED BY _____

JOB TITLE _____

DATE _____

Revision V

SECTION I

MANAGEMENT ELEMENTS
(45 POINTS)

IA. The Strategic Plan for Quality Improvement (11 Points)

It is virtually impossible to successfully implement Statistical Process Control (SPC) without a plan of action.

Does your strategic plan for quality improvement address the following?

	Yes	No
1. Management involvement/approval	___	___
2. Written quality policy	___	___
3. Quality manual development (i.e., revision)	___	___
4. SPC coordinator development (i.e., ongoing training, recertification)	___	___
5. Ongoing SPC training program	___	___
6. Utilization of quality costs/benefits analysis	___	___

	Yes	No
7. Identification of projects using SPC tools and techniques	___	___
8. Written preventive action procedures for process control	___	___
9. SPC utilization as a measure of performance and as a basis for recognition	___	___
10. Quality and cross-functional problem solving team meetings and schedule	___	___
11. Ongoing data collection and problem solving activities	___	___

VERIFICATION REQUIREMENTS:

To receive credit for Section IA, the following must accompany the PQR:

Submitted:

A current 12-month strategic plan signed and approved by management. _____

This plan shall include:
- Specific action items _____
- Designation of responsible individuals _____
- Proposed implementation/completion dates (MO/DY/YR) _____

IB. Quality Philosophy (4 Points)

First and foremost, SPC is a philosophy; a way of doing business. Therefore, upper management should provide the leadership toward adoption of this dramatic shift away from thinking that quality comes through inspection to quality through prevention. Leadership needs to be dynamic, aggressive, and above all else, tangible. The response by upper management to this section provides a clear indicator of their depth of commitment.

APPENDIX A

	Yes	No	N/A

1. Is there a published quality philosophy/policy statement on file? ____ ____

2. Which of the following is included in your quality policy?
   a. Philosophy of prevention ____ ____
   b. Reduction of quality costs ____ ____
   c. Continuous process improvement ____ ____
   d. Reduction of variation ____ ____
   e. Employee involvement ____ ____
   f. Management's responsibilities ____ ____
   g. Customer satisfaction ____ ____

3. Is your quality policy communicated to suppliers, customers, and internal personnel? ____ ____

4. Which of the following people have approved and signed your quality policy?
   a. CEO/president ____ ____ ____
   b. Plant/general manager ____ ____ ____
   c. Engineering manager ____ ____ ____
   d. Manufacturing engineering manager ____ ____ ____
   e. Production manager ____ ____ ____
   f. Quality manager ____ ____ ____
   g. Purchasing manager ____ ____ ____
   h. Finance manager ____ ____ ____
   i. SPC coordinator ____ ____ ____
   j. Other (specify) _____ ____ ____ ____

VERIFICATION REQUIREMENTS:

To receive credit for Section IB the following must be on file with the Supplier Quality Assistance Group (SQAG) at StorageTek or accompany the completed PQR.

	Submitted:	On File:
• A current quality policy	____	____
• Evidence of how the policy is communicated	____	____

IC. SPC Coordination/Management (10 Points)

Within an organization there should be one person who will provide management/administration of your SPC program. This individual should possess a variety of skills. This section concentrates on the most verifiable of those skills...**technical knowledge.** In addition it will help determine the extent to which the SPC coordinator's position is a viable one.

	Yes	No	N/A
1. Is there an SPC coordinator?	___	___	
2. Is the role of coordinator their sole function?	___	___	
3. Is the coordinator's position outside of the Quality department?	___	___	
4. Does the coordinator have more than 50 hours of any formal SPC training?	___	___	
5. Does the coordinator's training include theory, philosophy, concept of variation, capability analysis, control charting, basic problem solving techniques, Pareto and cause/effect diagram usage?	___	___	
6. Does the coordinator have formal training in advanced SPC and statistical problem solving techniques such as: active uses of control charts (both variable and attribute), the ranking method of cause/effect diagramming, and advanced problem solving techniques such as design of experiments?	___	___	
7. Is there a written job description for the coordinator's position?	___	___	
8. Would you be agreeable to your coordinator completing a confidential SPC skills evaluation?	___	___	
9. If your coordinator has taken the skills evaluation, was his/her score 75% or greater?	___	___	___
10. If your coordinator has taken the skills evaluation more than once, has there been improvement?	___	___	___

APPENDIX A

VERIFICATION REQUIREMENTS:

To receive credit for Section IC the following must be on file with the SQAG or accompany the completed PQR:

	Submitted:	On File:
• Job description for the person responsible for SPC coordination	_____	_____
• SPC coordinator skills evaluation	_____	_____

(Note: Answering "no" to question 8 will default questions 9 and 10 to a "no" answer.)

ID. Training (10 Points)

This section of the PQR determines the extent of your training program. It examines audiences targeted for training, length of courses, content material, etc.

Which groups, during the next 12 months, are included in your ongoing training schedule?

	Yes	No	N/A*	Dates (MO/DY/YR)	Hours
1. Inspectors	___	___	___	_____	___
2. Supervisors	___	___	___	_____	___
3. Operators	___	___	___	_____	___
4. Administration/support	___	___	___	_____	___
5. Management	___	___	___	_____	___
6. New employees	___	___	___	_____	___
7. Product/design/mfg. engineers	___	___	___	_____	___

Please indicate who will be providing the SPC instruction and the type of SPC instruction (i.e., CBT, classroom, etc.) in the space provided.

Have 75% of the people in each of the following groups received SPC training?

	%	Yes	No	N/A
8. Inspectors	___	___	___	___
9. Supervisors	___	___	___	___
10. Operators	___	___	___	___
11. Administration/support	___	___	___	___
12. Management	___	___	___	___
13. Product/design/manufacturing engineers	___	___	___	___
14. Are you utilizing an SPC training manual?		___	___	
15. Is your training linked to projects?		___	___	

*If N/A, please explain after each question.

Which of the following elements are included in your training program?

	Yes	No
16. Philosophy (prevention vs. detection)	___	___
17. Concept of reducing variation	___	___
18. Histogram (construction and interpretation)	___	___
19. Capability (concepts and assessment)	___	___
20. Control charting (theory and construction)	___	___
21. Control charting (analysis and interpretation)	___	___
22. Other statistical charting tools (short run, attribute, EWMA, etc.)	___	___
23. Implementation (flow charting, action planning, goal setting, etc.)	___	___
24. Problem solving (Pareto, cause/effect, etc.)	___	___
25. Advanced problem solving (regression analysis, D.O.E., hypothesis testing, ANOVA, etc.)	___	___

> VERIFICATION REQUIREMENTS:
>
> To receive credit for Section ID the following must be on file or accompany the completed PQR:
>
>   Submitted: On-file:
>
> - A current 12-month schedule for training complete with participants
> - A copy of your current training materials
> - A copy of your course syllabus
> - An outline of projects linked to training

IE. Economic Considerations of Quality (5 Points)

Cost reductions and other cost benefits of quality improvement are essential to determine success, identify project areas, and stimulate continuous improvement. Although some cost benefits are difficult to quantify, this should not preclude the use of specific cost data to identify where resources are being wasted as well as where cost reductions have resulted from SPC implementation. It is important to recognize economic considerations for quality may be demonstrated through various metrics (i.e., labor hours, percentages, etc.). This section highlights areas which include 1) management and coordination of a quality cost accounting system, and 2) criteria for cost analysis.

	Yes	No
1. Is analysis of quality costs/benefits utilized at your facility?		
2. Is the information regarding quality costs/benefits disseminated throughout all levels of management?		
3. Does your facility break down quality costs/benefits information into the following categories?		
Prevention		
Appraisal		
Internal failures		
External failures		

	Yes	No	N/A

4. Are costs associated with the following measured and tracked? (Prevention)
    - Quality planning
    - Process control elements
    - Development of quality systems
    - Equipment training
    - Product design verification
    - Quality systems management
    - Preventive maintenance
    - Housekeeping
    - First article inspection
    - Capital equipment
    - Supplier qualification program
    - Other (specify)_____

5. Are the costs/benefits associated with the following areas measured and tracked? (Appraisal)
    - Receiving/source inspection
    - In-process inspection
    - Final inspection
    - Calibration/maintenance of test/ inspection equipment
    - Quality audits
    - Product test
    - Outside lab evaluation
    - Life testing
    - Other (specify)_____

6. Are the costs/benefits associated with the following areas measured and tracked? (Internal Failure)
    - Scrap
    - Rework
    - Material review
    - Design failure
    - Down time
    - Failure analysis
    - Re-test
    - Engineering changes
    - Tooling repair/modification
    - Other (specify)_____

APPENDIX A

7. Are the costs/benefits associated with the following areas measured and tracked? (External Failure)   <u>Yes</u>   <u>No</u>   <u>N/A</u>
   - Warranty charges
   - Field evaluation and testing
   - Product liability
   - Insurance
   - Premium freight costs
   - Responding to customer complaints
   - Customer service
   - Return expenses
   - Product recall
   - Other (specify)_____

8. Are the costs/benefits associated with the following areas measured and tracked?
   - Sales
   - Market share
   - Repeat buys
   - Customer base
   - Other (specify)_____

9. Is there a breakdown of quality costs/benefits by specific area (i.e., product line, assembly area, and/or machine center)?

10. Have process improvement projects been identified through the use of quality costs/benefits analysis?

VERIFICATION REQUIREMENTS:

To receive credit for Section IE the following must accompany the PQR:

                                                                       Submitted:

Dated examples demonstrating the active use of quality costs/benefits analysis including:
- Identification of specific areas of application (product line, manufacturing cell, etc.)
- Identification of quality improvement projects (including rationale)
- Management involvement

These examples shall be itemized under each area (i.e., prevention, appraisal, internal failure and external failure).

(Note: Any information deemed proprietary in the quality costs/benefits analysis may be blackened or obliterated.)

IF. Employee Involvement (5 Points)

It is critical that all employees adopt the philosophy of SPC for the ongoing success of implementation. For employees to have ownership in the active use of SPC, it must be linked to tangible incentives (i.e., bonuses, awards, etc.).

	Yes	No
1. Is SPC utilization included as part of the job description for personnel who have been trained in SPC?	___	___
2. Is SPC utilization included as part of the job description for all personnel?	___	___
3. Is SPC utilization part of the performance review for personnel who have been trained in SPC?	___	___
4. Is SPC utilization part of the performance review for all personnel?	___	___
5. Is there some type of remuneration for quality improvement related activities (individuals or teams)?	___	___

VERIFICATION REQUIREMENTS:

To receive credit for Section IF the following must be on file with the SQAG or accompany the completed PQR:

	Submitted:	On File:
• A copy of a job description from someone outside of the quality department	___	___
• A copy of a performance review from someone outside of the quality department	___	___
• A description of the type of remuneration for the use of quality improvement related activities	___	___

(Note: No credit will be given for question 1 or 3 if no training has occurred.)

SECTION II

OPERATIONS
(55 POINTS)

IIA. Process Improvement Project (10 Points)

A project should identify an element in your processes (i.e., manufacturing, service, support, etc.) Once a project is successfully completed, that success can be used as a catalyst for expanded SPC implementation within the facility.

<u>Yes</u>   <u>No</u>

1. Has a process improvement project utilizing SPC methodologies, including cross-functional problem solving teams, been started in the last 12 months? ____ ____

2. Does the project identify an end product parameter, in-process product parameter or a process parameter in your manufacturing/support operations as a candidate for continuous improvement? ____ ____

3. Have quality costs/benefits been used to establish a baseline from which a return on investment can be determined? ____ ____

4. Were quantifiable goals for cost reduction/quality improvement set? ____ ____

5. Have these goals been met for this project or for projects completed in the previous 12 months? ____ ____

VERIFICATION REQUIREMENTS:

To receive credit for Section IIA the following must accompany the completed PQR:

<u>Submitted:</u>

- Description of the SPC project and identification of the process _____
- StorageTek part numbers affected by this process _____
- Names and positions of the problem solving team members _____
- Associated analysis of quality costs/benefits _____
- A list of set project goals and results achieved _____

IIB. Data Collection (20 Points)

While data collection is only part of process control, it is a vital cog in the improvement of any process. This section deals with the tools used and the extent of their use.

	Yes	No

1. What percent of StorageTek products have capability studies being calculated on an ongoing basis?
    0 – 9% _____
    10 – 25% _____
    26 – 50% _____
    51 – 75% _____
    76 – 100% _____

2. Do the majority of parameters measured on those parts have capability indices (Cpk) as follows?
    Greater than or equal to 2.00 _____
    Between 1.33 and 1.99 _____
    Less than 1.33 _____

3. What percent of measurable operations/processes/machines have utilized variable process control charting methods?
    0 – 9% _____
    10 – 25% _____
    26 – 50% _____
    51 – 75% _____
    76 – 100% _____

4. What percent of attribute parameters have utilized attribute control charting methods?
    0 – 49% _____
    50 – 100% _____

5. Is data being collected during operations, rather than taken solely from inspection history (i.e., on-line, real time)? _____ _____

6. Are changes and actions to the process being continuously documented on the control charts used during data collection (i.e., shift changes, equipment changes, operator changes, etc.)? _____ _____

VERIFICATION REQUIREMENTS:

To receive credit for Section IIB the following must be on file with the SQAG or accompany the completed PQR:

	Submitted:	On File:
• Number of StorageTek parts with open POs and associated data capability studies	_____	
• Graphic detailed production flow charts identifying the parameters/operations where capability studies and control charting are being used for each part number or process	_____	_____
• Dated copies of the capability studies and control charts identified on the flow charts	_____	
• Control charts demonstrating active use of the note section (i.e., log sheets)	_____	

IIC. Problem Solving (25 Points)

SPC IS NOT JUST DATA COLLECTION. Without positive answers to questions in this section your data collection is worthless. The problem solving tools run the gamut from the simple (e.g., histogram analysis) to the complex (e.g., fractional factorial experiments). Section IIC also determines the management of your problem solving activities.

	Yes	No
1. Which of the following basic tools have been used to continually reduce variation within the last 12 months?		
a. Capability studies	_____	_____
b. Variable control charts	_____	_____
c. Other charting methods	_____	_____
d. Pareto analysis	_____	_____
2. Have you employed factorial design of experiments to reduce variation/manufacturing costs in the last 12 months?	_____	_____

	Yes	No

3. Have you realized a quantifiable quality improvement/cost reduction from your design of experiments? _____ _____

4. Does your quality manual or written preventive action procedure specify the process to be followed when a capability index (Cpk) is less than 1.33 and where the process shows lack of control? _____ _____

5. Which of the following meetings are held on a continuous basis at your facility to promote continuous improvement?

   a. Problem solving meetings where capability is insufficient (Cpk < 1.33) or where the process shows lack of control _____ _____

   b. Process control steering committee meetings for SPC implementation _____ _____

   c. Weekly operator/supervisor/management meetings to review process successes/failures _____ _____

   d. Semi-annual communication meetings where upper management recognizes outstanding performances _____ _____

   e. Action plan review/revision meetings _____ _____

VERIFICATION REQUIREMENTS:

To receive credit for Section IIC the following must be on file or accompany the completed PQR:

	Submitted:	On File:
• Before and after copies of the basic tools referencing the corrective action taken to reduce variation	_____	
• A copy of the experimental design, method of analysis, and an explanation of the quality improvement/cost reduction achieved	_____	
• Copies of problem solving meeting minutes/notes identifying the problem(s) addressed and the corrective action taken to improve process capability or consistency	_____	
• A copy of the preventive action procedure which outlines the requirements for formal problem solving	_____	_____
• Copies of minutes/agenda for all other indicated meetings	_____	

SCORING SYSTEM

PREFACE

Appendix A deals with the scoring of the PQR. Each section will be worth a specified number of points. A percentage will be calculated and matched to that number of points per section. For example, if you answered yes to 15 out of 18 questions in a section worth 20 points, then:

$15/18 = .83$, or 83% of $20 = 16.7$.

You would be awarded 16.7 points for that section. A perfect score would be 100. Points will not be awarded until verification is confirmed by the user.

Point Allocation:

SECTION	DESCRIPTION	POINTS
I	MANAGEMENT ELEMENTS	
	A. Strategic Plan	11
	B. Quality Policy-Philosophy	4
	C. SPC Coordinator/Management	10
	D. Training	10
	E. Economic Considerations of Quality	5
	F. Employee Involvement	5
	Total:	45
II	OPERATIONS	
	A. Process Improvement Project	10
	B. Data Collection	20
	C. Problem Solving	25
	Total:	55

Section IIB

Questions 1 & 3

PERCENT	POINTS
0 – 9%	0
10 – 25%	1
26 – 50%	2
51 – 75%	3
76 – 100%	4

Question 2

INDEX (Cpk)	POINTS
Less than 1.33	0
Between 1.33 and 1.99	3
Greater than or equal to 2.00	5

Question 4

PERCENT	POINTS
0 – 49%	0
50 – 100%	1

Question 5   1 point

Question 6   5 points

Section IIC

Question 1   2 points for each tool

Question 2   5 points

Questions 3 & 4   3 points each

Question 5   A   2 points
                     B-E 1 point

APPENDIX B

World Class Health Care versus Medical Tradition: Two Case Studies

World Class Health Care requires a thorough diagnosis and coordinated team action. Flow charting, a statistical tool, optimizes communication between treatment team members. It assures an accurate, thorough diagnostic and treatment process.

Statistical Process Control charts improve the treatment team's ability to monitor and control drug therapy. All team members (physician, psychologist, nurse educator, and patient) must have access to all statistical data.

The following case study was documented and diagrammed by Rosanne D. Gingrich, MD, for Quality Health Systems of America, Inc. Acknowledgment is given to Dr. Gingrich and Quality Health Systems of America, Inc. for permission to use this case study.

Case:

A 61-year-old Hispanic male was brought to the emergency room (ER) by ambulance in full cardiac arrest. He had been found unresponsive at home in bed at approximately 0700.

He had a history of insulin-dependent diabetes mellitus and hypertension. He was cyanotic, pulseless, and apneic. He was asystolic on cardiac monitor. Full ACLS (Advanced Cardiac Life Support) protocols were followed; patient remained asystolic and was pronounced dead at 0827. His daughter, after viewing the body, tearfully accused the ER physician of "not trying hard enough."

Previous hospital admission records revealed two outpatient procedures for photocoagulation of the retina for diabetic proliferative retinopathy. A phone call to his doctor provoked the comments that the patient was "noncompliant" and had "bad disease."

The wife related that her husband had started to feel ill the previous afternoon after he had been exposed to truck exhaust fumes while setting up tables for a flea market.

On the way home from the flea market he complained of feeling nauseated and kept the car window open on the way home. He did not complain of chest pain. He refused to go to the emergency room. On arrival home, he seemed to feel better.

He ate dinner and seemed comfortable. His wife stated that he did spend a restless night. He got up at 0400, watched some TV, then returned to bed at 0600. She said his blood pressure was "always high" and his medications were insulin plus Corgard (a beta-blocker) and chlorthalidone (a thiazide diuretic) for his hypertension.

The daughter, while being consoled by friends, mumbled something about her father's drinking.

Autopsy report showed arteriosclerosis of the aorta plus left ventricular hypertrophy (enlarged heart). Probable cause of death was cardiac arrythmia.

Compared Approach: Medical Tradition Versus Quality Protocol

The quality approach to this man and his family differs significantly from Medical Tradition.

> Medical Tradition presumes that hypertension is a random occurrence. It assumes that the origin, the genesis, of the disease is organic. Treatment for high blood pressure is considered to be a routine task for medication.

> Medical Tradition presumes diabetes mellitus is a complex disease caused by genetics or physiology.

Under our current system, the patient comes to the doctor's office with a problem. The problem described in this case is diagnosed and labeled as "insulin-dependent diabetes mellitus" or "essential hypertension" (high blood pressure).

The patient is given a prescription. He is advised not to drink alcohol in excess, to stop smoking, and to watch his diet. The diabetes and hypertension are monitored at the patient's discretion.

> Quality health care givers make no presumptions or assumptions about the occurrence or causes of disease. The genesis of disease may or may not be random. The root cause may or may not be organic.

Quality health care protocols are distinguished by three characteristics.

1. A complete history is always collected. The diagnosis is in the history: physical, behavioral, and psychological. Data must be collected and graphed in the sequence and order in which it occurs.
2. Process improvement plans are guided by and monitored using statistical method from the viewpoint of quality control. Flow diagrams, fishbone diagrams, Pareto charts, and control charts are all used.
3. All members of the treatment team (physician, psychologist, nurse educator, and patient) have equal access to medical record data. All share responsibility for outcome and cost.

Diabetes and hypertension are outputs of a process. Neither is a random occurrence. Lifestyle, thoughts, emotions, and physiology are all probable root causes.

The process must be fully diagnosed using a thorough scientific analysis of the patient's history. A simple fishbone diagram (Figure B.1) starts the analysis:

Medical Tradition takes action based on a single data point of output, a high blood pressure reading or a high blood sugar chemistry reading. Because the process (the system of chance causes which is responsible for the output) is not improved, diabetes and high blood pressure will continue to be produced.

Therefore, disease not health, is the manufactured product.

Treatment taken without regard to the patient's statistical state of control is tampering. Tampering causes chaos. Chaos ruins quality.

Quality protocols provide structure and discipline. Quality standards are established using statistical methods from the viewpoint of quality control. Team expertise (physician, psychologist, nurse educator, and patient) is used to evaluate the process. The team establishes process improvement priorities. Control action is taken by the patient. Process output is analyzed using control charts to document the evolution of a constantly improving process.

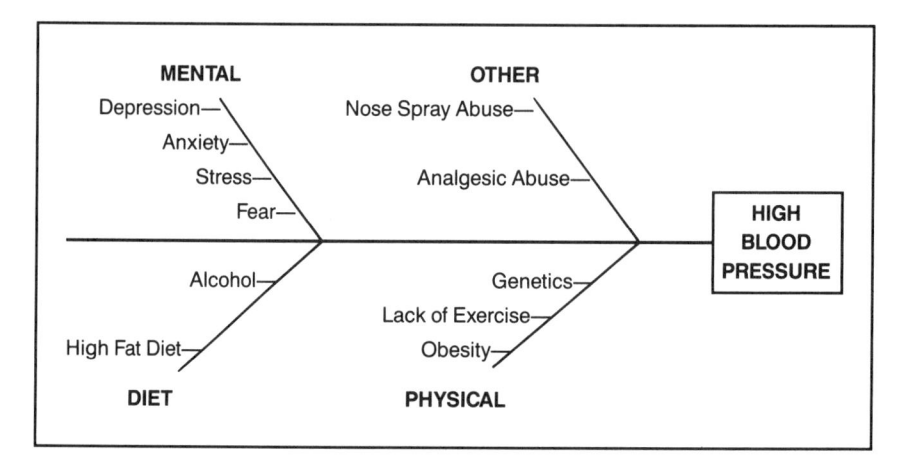

```
                MENTAL                  OTHER
         Depression─╲          Nose Spray Abuse─╲
           Anxiety─╲
            Stress─╲            Analgesic Abuse─╲
              Fear─╲                                    ┌──────────┐
                    ╲                                   │   HIGH   │
─────────────────────┴───────────────────────────┬──────│  BLOOD   │
                    ╱                            │      │ PRESSURE │
            Alcohol─╱             Genetics─╱            └──────────┘
                             Lack of Exercise─╱
      High Fat Diet─╱              Obesity─╱
                 DIET                 PHYSICAL
```

Figure B.1 Scientific analysis begins with fishbone diagram.

This sample quality protocol (Figure B.2) graphically displays the process which must be followed for the diagnosis and treatment of high blood pressure. It was developed by an emergency medicine physician, an internal medicine specialist, a health educator, and a psychologist. A medical librarian provided essential research support services.

Group consensus is used to approve policy. Experience, published scientific research, and quality control data prompt protocol revisions.

Walking Through a Quality Protocol for Hypertension

First the physician determines whether the high blood pressure is a crisis which demands immediate medical intervention. (See flow chart (Figure B.2) for treatment of hypertensive emergencies and toxemia of pregnancy.)

If the high blood pressure is not an emergency, blood pressure readings are taken four times a day. Readings would be made at four-hour intervals while the patient is awake, for six consecutive days. Blood pressure readings would be recorded on a chart by the patient and the nurse educator.

Lifestyle, emotional, and psychological factors must be assessed using the Michigan Alcohol Screening Test, the Beck Depression Inventory, the Center for Disease Control's computerized health risk appraisal, and the Holmes and Rahe Social Readjustment Rating Scale.

Hypertension can be caused or aggravated by medications. A complete history of medication use and abuse would uncover use of nose spray, analgesics, steroids, thyroid medication, antidepressants, or other drugs which affect blood pressure.

APPENDIX B

QUALITY PROTOCOL FOR HIGH BLOOD PRESSURE
QUALITY HEALTH SYSTEMS OF AMERICA, INC.

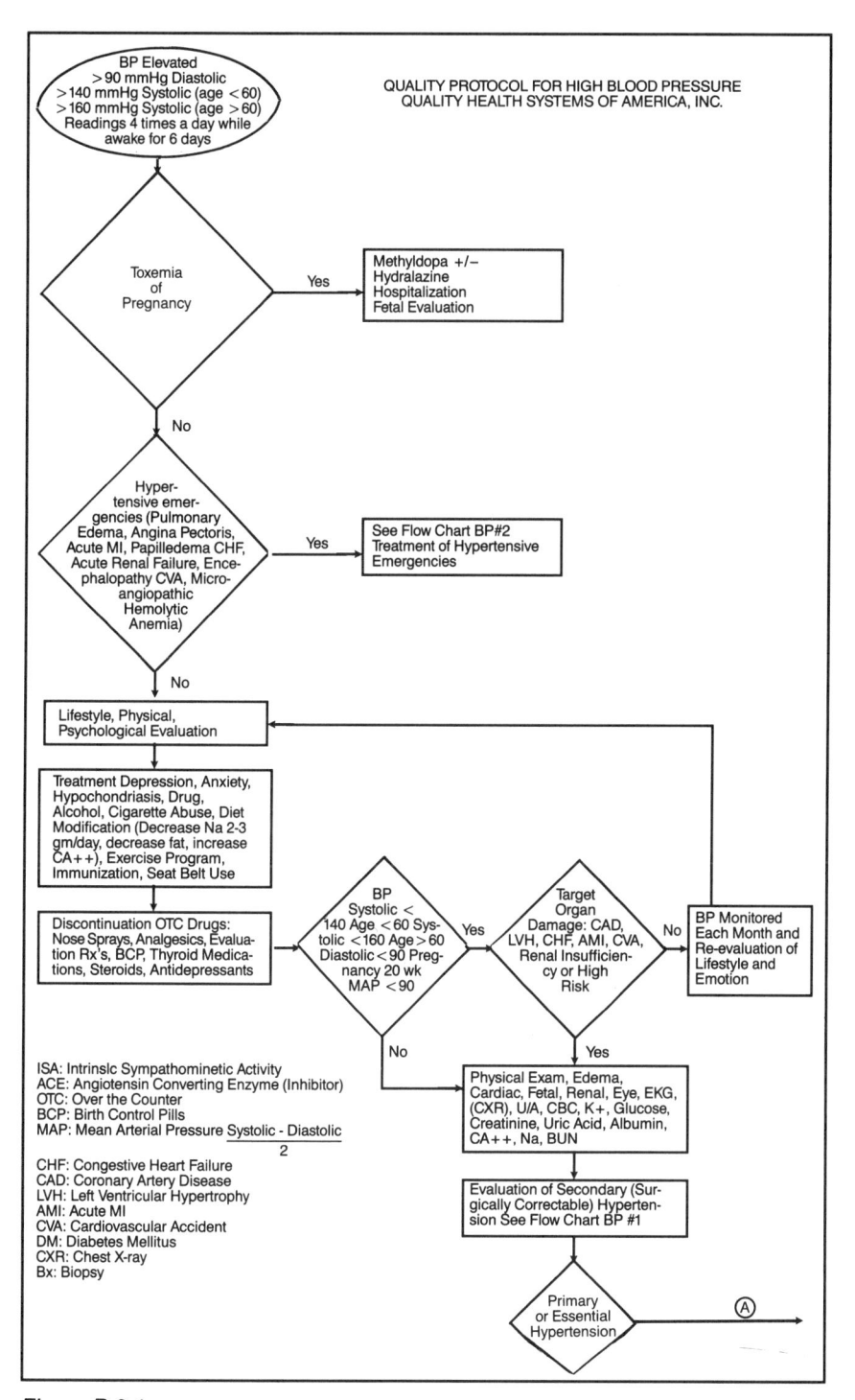

```
                    ┌─────────────────────┐
                    │    BP Elevated      │
                    │ >90 mmHg Diastolic  │
                    │>140 mmHg Systolic   │
                    │   (age <60)         │
                    │>160 mmHg Systolic   │
                    │   (age >60)         │
                    │ Readings 4 times a  │
                    │ day while awake     │
                    │     for 6 days      │
                    └──────────┬──────────┘
                               │
                    ┌──────────▼──────────┐       ┌──────────────────────┐
                    │     Toxemia of      │  Yes  │ Methyldopa +/−       │
                    │     Pregnancy       ├──────▶│ Hydralazine          │
                    │                     │       │ Hospitalization      │
                    └──────────┬──────────┘       │ Fetal Evaluation     │
                               │ No               └──────────────────────┘
                    ┌──────────▼──────────┐
                    │   Hypertensive      │
                    │   emergencies       │       ┌──────────────────────┐
                    │ (Pulmonary Edema,   │  Yes  │ See Flow Chart BP#2  │
                    │ Angina Pectoris,    ├──────▶│ Treatment of         │
                    │ Acute MI, Papill-   │       │ Hypertensive         │
                    │ edema CHF, Acute    │       │ Emergencies          │
                    │ Renal Failure,      │       └──────────────────────┘
                    │ Encephalopathy CVA, │
                    │ Microangiopathic    │
                    │ Hemolytic Anemia)   │
                    └──────────┬──────────┘
                               │ No
                    ┌──────────▼──────────────────┐
                    │ Lifestyle, Physical,        │◀─────────────────────┐
                    │ Psychological Evaluation    │                      │
                    └──────────┬──────────────────┘                      │
                    ┌──────────▼──────────────────┐                      │
                    │ Treatment Depression,       │                      │
                    │ Anxiety, Hypochondriasis,   │                      │
                    │ Drug, Alcohol, Cigarette    │                      │
                    │ Abuse, Diet Modification    │                      │
                    │ (Decrease Na 2-3 gm/day,    │                      │
                    │ decrease fat, increase      │                      │
                    │ CA++), Exercise Program,    │                      │
                    │ Immunization, Seat Belt Use │                      │
                    └──────────┬──────────────────┘                      │
                               │                                         │
                    ┌──────────▼──────────────┐  ┌────────────┐  ┌──────────────┐
                    │ Discontinuation OTC     │  │    BP      │  │ Target Organ │
                    │ Drugs: Nose Sprays,     │  │ Systolic < │  │ Damage: CAD, │
                    │ Analgesics, Evaluation  │  │ 140 Age<60 │  │ LVH, CHF,    │  No  ┌─────────────┐
                    │ Rx's, BCP, Thyroid      │  │ Systolic < │◀─│ AMI, CVA,    ├─────▶│ BP Monitored│
                    │ Medications, Steroids,  │  │ 160 Age>60 │Yes│ Renal Insuf- │      │ Each Month  │
                    │ Antidepressants         │  │ Diastolic  │  │ ficiency or  │      │ and Re-     │
                    └─────────────────────────┘  │ <90 Preg-  │  │ High Risk    │      │ evaluation  │
                                                 │ nancy 20wk │  └──────┬───────┘      │ of Lifestyle│
                                                 │ MAP <90    │         │Yes           │ and Emotion │
                                                 └──────┬─────┘         │              └─────────────┘
                                                        │No             ▼
                                                        │       ┌──────────────────────┐
                                                        │       │ Physical Exam, Edema,│
                                                        │       │ Cardiac, Fetal,      │
                                                        │       │ Renal, Eye, EKG,     │
                                                        │       │ (CXR), U/A, CBC, K+, │
                                                        │       │ Glucose, Creatinine, │
                                                        │       │ Uric Acid, Albumin,  │
                                                        │       │ CA++, Na, BUN        │
                                                        │       └──────────┬───────────┘
                                                        │                  │
                                                        │       ┌──────────▼───────────┐
                                                        │       │ Evaluation of        │
                                                        │       │ Secondary (Surgically│
                                                        │       │ Correctable) Hyper-  │
                                                        │       │ tension See Flow     │
                                                        │       │ Chart BP #1          │
                                                        │       └──────────┬───────────┘
                                                        │                  │
                                                        │       ┌──────────▼───────────┐
                                                        │       │     Primary or       │
                                                        │       │     Essential        ├──▶ (A)
                                                        │       │     Hypertension     │
                                                        │       └──────────────────────┘
```

ISA: Intrinsic Sympathominetic Activity
ACE: Angiotensin Converting Enzyme (Inhibitor)
OTC: Over the Counter
BCP: Birth Control Pills
MAP: Mean Arterial Pressure $\frac{\text{Systolic} - \text{Diastolic}}{2}$
CHF: Congestive Heart Failure
CAD: Coronary Artery Disease
LVH: Left Ventricular Hypertrophy
AMI: Acute MI
CVA: Cardiovascular Accident
DM: Diabetes Mellitus
CXR: Chest X-ray
Bx: Biopsy

Figure B.2.1

A Pareto analysis would summarize the data. The statistical picture helps the team identify the vital few causes which are probably responsible for the diabetes and high blood pressure. Output indicators (high blood pressure readings or high blood sugar chemistry results) would be monitored using control charts to document process improvements.

In this case smoking cessation and treatment for alcoholism would be priorities. Dietary modifications and exercise would be secondary.

Three weeks later, the patient and his family would have a better understanding of diabetes and hypertension. Smoking cessation and abstinence from alcohol would have lowered the patient's blood pressure slightly. Abstinence would have aided in insulin stabilization.

The patient's blood pressure may not yet be in control, according to the control chart. Diabetes complicates the elevated blood pressure. Drinking habits complicate treatment. Hence, a physical examination would be required. Some blood studies, a urinalysis, an EKG, and a possible chest X-ray may be necessary to evaluate the secondary causes of hypertension.

For this walk-through we have assumed the physician or a physician assistant team member determines there is no difference in the blood pressure readings taken in the arms or legs. Femoral pulses are normal and the patient has no sudden onset of pain in the calves while walking. There are no turbulent flow sounds over the renal arteries. The onset of hypertension has been slow; there are no spells of nervousness, headache, sweating, or large swings in blood pressure readings.

The patient does not feel weak. Serum creatinine and urinalysis results are normal. The physician or physician assistant concludes the elevated BP is "essential" or primary hypertension.

Only now would pharmacologic treatment be started. Drug treatment would be individualized with emphasis on age, race, and risk factors. Clinical memory is no substitute for a diagrammed protocol.

Because this patient has diabetes mellitus, the best choices for therapy are angiotensin converting enzyme (ACE) inhibitors or calcium channel blockers. Using the flow diagrammed quality protocol, the team chooses 10 mg of lisinopril a day. Blood pressure must be monitored by the patient. Readings must be charted on a control chart.

Systolic and diastolic control limits are set after considering the patient's age, sex, race, and any known organ damage (Figure B.3).

In our case study, reevaluation by the team occurs every two weeks. Lifestyle and emotional process factors are scrutinized.

If the blood pressure remains out of control the dose of ACE inhibitor is increased slowly to the maximum recommended. If blood pressure remains out of control, a calcium channel blocker is substituted for the ACE inhibitor.

APPENDIX B

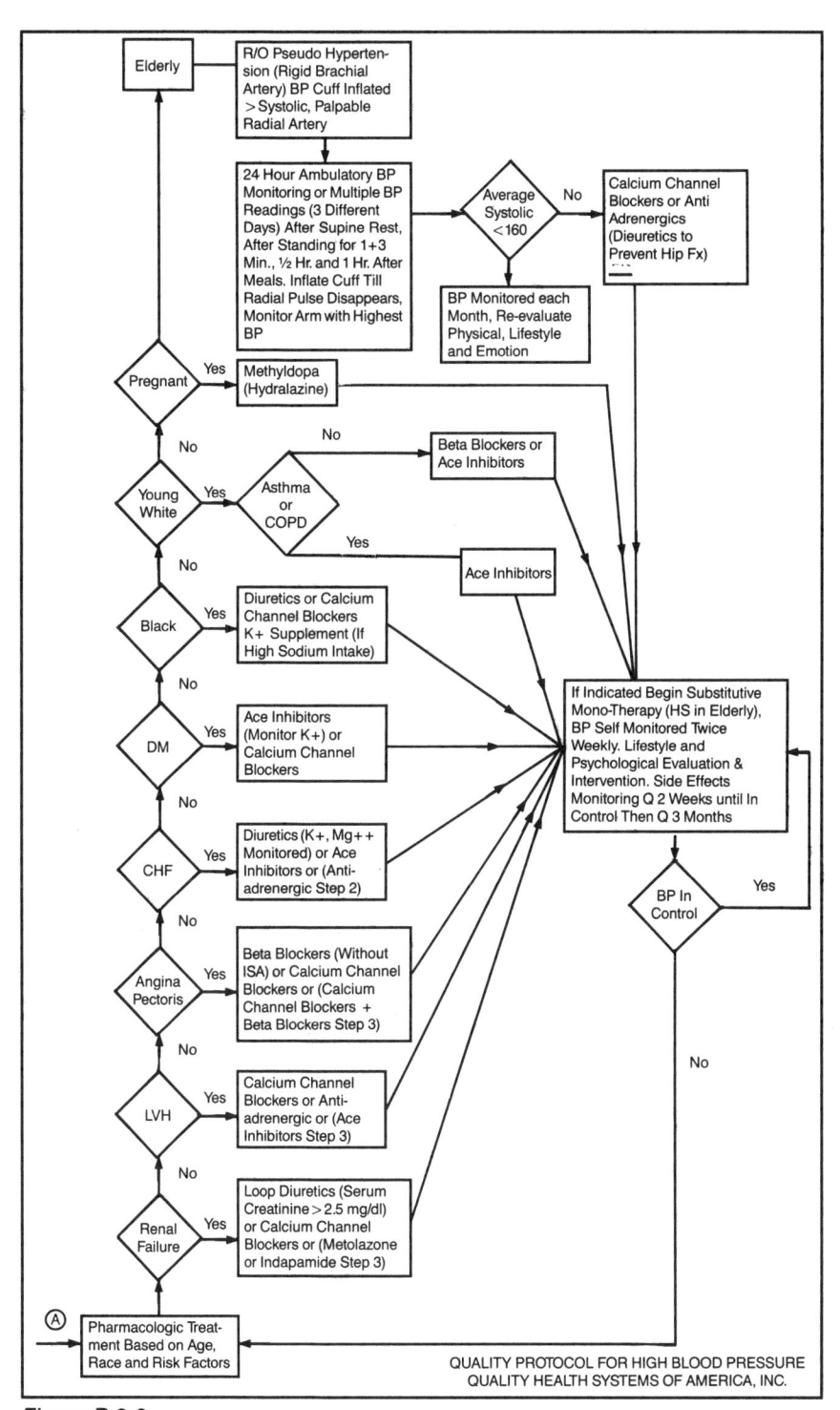

Figure B.2.2 — QUALITY PROTOCOL FOR HIGH BLOOD PRESSURE, QUALITY HEALTH SYSTEMS OF AMERICA, INC.

Elderly: R/O Pseudo Hypertension (Rigid Brachial Artery) BP Cuff Inflated > Systolic, Palpable Radial Artery → 24 Hour Ambulatory BP Monitoring or Multiple BP Readings (3 Different Days) After Supine Rest, After Standing for 1+3 Min., ½ Hr. and 1 Hr. After Meals. Inflate Cuff Till Radial Pulse Disappears, Monitor Arm with Highest BP

- Average Systolic < 160?
  - **No** → Calcium Channel Blockers or Anti Adrenergics (Diuretics to Prevent Hip Fx)
  - **Yes** → BP Monitored each Month, Re-evaluate Physical, Lifestyle and Emotion

Pregnant: Yes → Methyldopa (Hydralazine)

Young White: Yes → Asthma or COPD?
  - No → Beta Blockers or Ace Inhibitors
  - Yes → Ace Inhibitors

Black: Yes → Diuretics or Calcium Channel Blockers K+ Supplement (If High Sodium Intake)

DM: Yes → Ace Inhibitors (Monitor K+) or Calcium Channel Blockers

CHF: Yes → Diuretics (K+, Mg++ Monitored) or Ace Inhibitors or (Anti-adrenergic Step 2)

Angina Pectoris: Yes → Beta Blockers (Without ISA) or Calcium Channel Blockers or (Calcium Channel Blockers + Beta Blockers Step 3)

LVH: Yes → Calcium Channel Blockers or Anti-adrenergic or (Ace Inhibitors Step 3)

Renal Failure: Yes → Loop Diuretics (Serum Creatinine > 2.5 mg/dl) or Calcium Channel Blockers or (Metolazone or Indapamide Step 3)

(A) Pharmacologic Treatment Based on Age, Race and Risk Factors

If Indicated Begin Substitutive Mono-Therapy (HS in Elderly), BP Self Monitored Twice Weekly. Lifestyle and Psychological Evaluation & Intervention. Side Effects Monitoring Q 2 Weeks until In Control Then Q 3 Months

BP In Control? Yes → (exit); No → (loop back)

176 THE QUALITY REVOLUTION AND HEALTH CARE

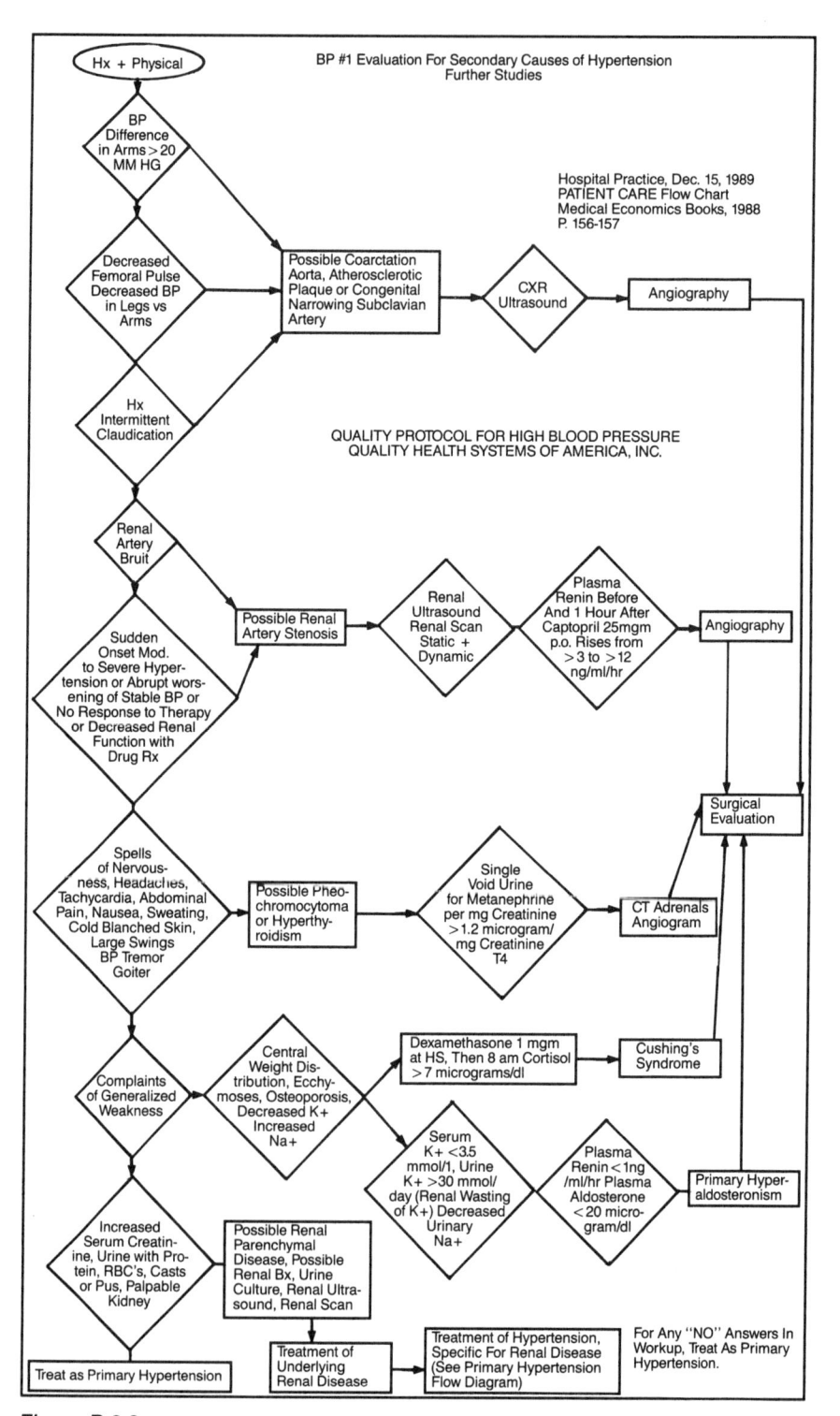

BP #1 Evaluation For Secondary Causes of Hypertension
Further Studies

Hospital Practice, Dec. 15, 1989
PATIENT CARE Flow Chart
Medical Economics Books, 1988
P. 156-157

QUALITY PROTOCOL FOR HIGH BLOOD PRESSURE
QUALITY HEALTH SYSTEMS OF AMERICA, INC.

For Any "NO" Answers In Workup, Treat As Primary Hypertension.

Figure B.2.3

APPENDIX B   177

BP #2 Treatment of Hypertensive Emergencies

QUALITY PROTOCOL FOR HIGH BLOOD PRESSURE
QUALITY HEALTH SYSTEMS OF AMERICA, INC.

Hypertensive Emergency → Pheochromocytoma → Alpha Blockade with Phentolamine or Prazosin or Labetalol (Alpha and Beta Blockade)

↓

Scleroderma with Renal Crisis → ACE Inhibitors or Labetalol

↓

Adrenergic Crisis Due to Amphetamine, its Analogs, Cocaine or MAO Inhibitor /Tyramine Syndrome → Labetalol or Combined Alpha & Beta Blockers

↓

Dissecting Aneurysm → Labetalol Plus Vasodilator or Gaglionic Blocker

↓

Malignant Phase of Essential Hypertension → Nitroprusside or Nifedipine or Labetalol or ACE Inhibitor + Furosemide

↓

Hypertension with Ischemic Heart Disease → Heart Rate >110 → IV NTG or Nitroprusside / Beta Blocker or Verapamil

↓

Severe Hypertension with Pulmonary Congestion → Signs of Poor Perfusion Clammy Skin, Decreased Mentation, Decreased Urine OutPut → Dobutamine Plus NTG or Nitroprusside / Furosemide IV or ACE Inhibitor (Enalapril IV)

↓

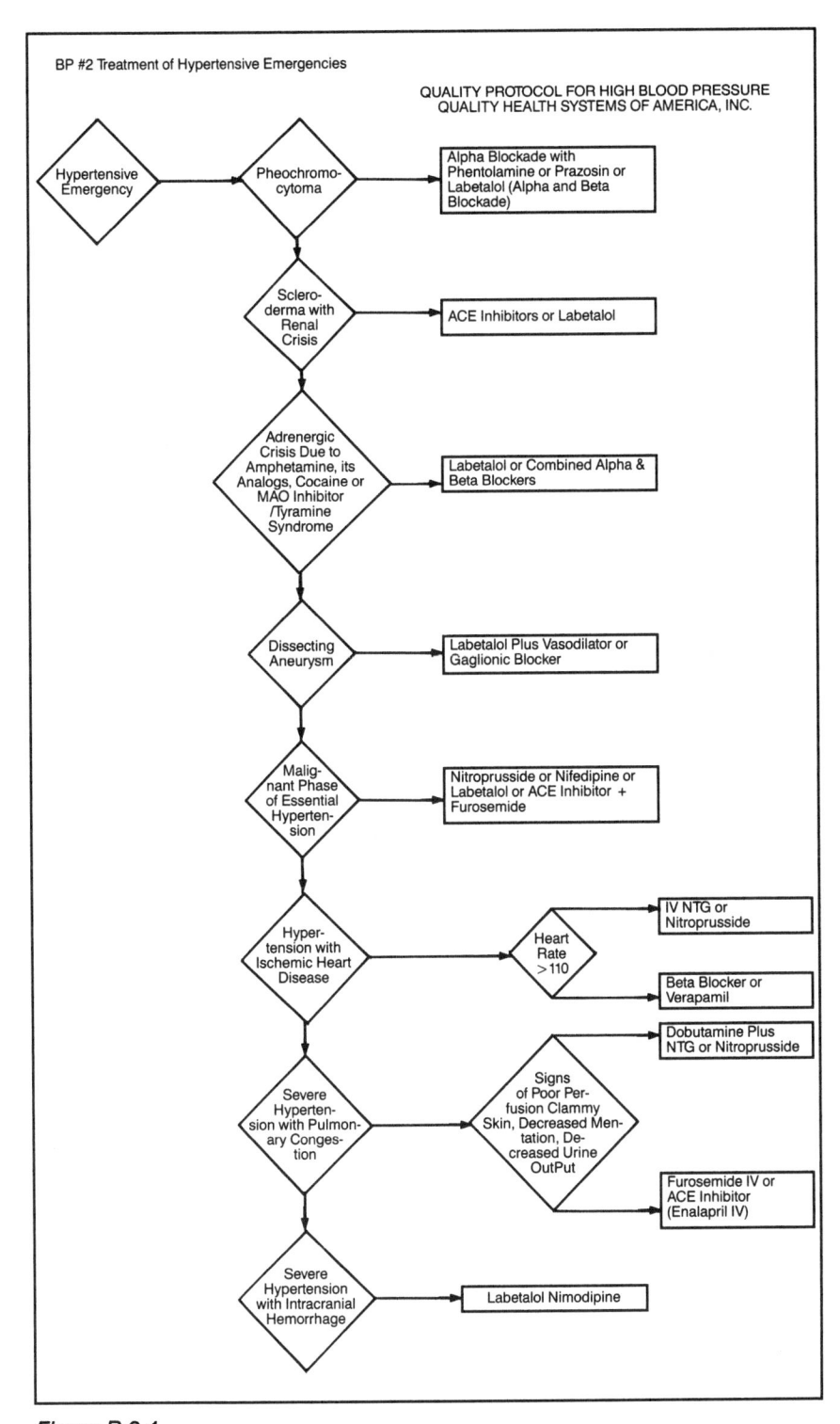

Severe Hypertension with Intracranial Hemorrhage → Labetalol Nimodipine

Figure B.2.4

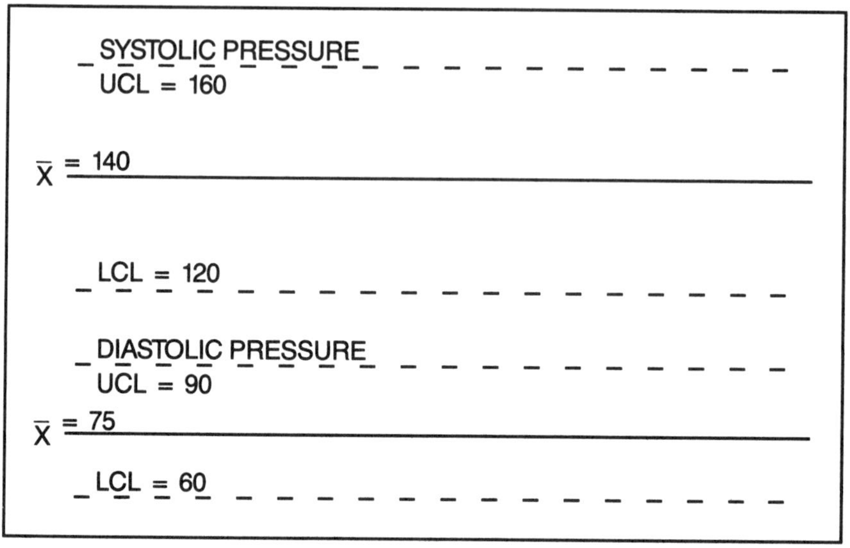

```
  SYSTOLIC PRESSURE
  UCL = 160   ─ ─ ─ ─ ─ ─ ─ ─ ─ ─ ─ ─

X̄ = 140
  ─────────────────────────────────

  LCL = 120   ─ ─ ─ ─ ─ ─ ─ ─ ─ ─ ─ ─

  DIASTOLIC PRESSURE
  UCL = 90    ─ ─ ─ ─ ─ ─ ─ ─ ─ ─ ─ ─

X̄ = 75
  ─────────────────────────────────

  LCL = 60    ─ ─ ─ ─ ─ ─ ─ ─ ─ ─ ─ ─
```

Figure B.3 Systolic and diastolic control limits are set.

Another Teaching Example

The following urine output, systolic and diastolic pressure control charts (Figures B.4 and B.5) were constructed using actual data from a 70-year-old Hispanic male in an intensive care unit.

The patient was receiving dopamine, Inacor, and Bretyllium. Dopamine, a drug which increases the perfusion of blood through the kidneys, also raises systolic blood pressure. Each drug output should have been monitored separately. (Although multiple doses of varying drugs are commonly prescribed, it is impossible to predict the consequences of simultaneously administered drugs.)

We graphed the known outputs of dopamine, systolic blood pressure, and urine output. Dopamine is administered intravenously by a machine which controls the flow of the drug. When the dose is adjusted a change in the output of the drug can be measured almost immediately. We graphed diastolic pressure because the raw data was available.

Urine measurements were recorded on the hour (Figures B.4 and B.5). Pressure samples were taken at half-hour intervals (Figure B.4).

The variation displayed on the urine output individual's chart indicates a number of special causes. The urine output was adequate enough to justify a smaller dose of dopamine. When the dopamine was decreased at 2100 an unusual increase in urine output was documented. The urine output process shifted again over the next four hours.

Statistical process control could have added the important elements of precision and accuracy to this drug therapy.

The variation found on the average moving range chart of the patient's systolic blood pressure indicates a special cause. In addition, the first 12 hours of mean systolic pressure readings, 174, was too high. The high systolic pressure was probably related to the administration of dopamine.

Statistical method from the viewpoint of quality control would have alerted the nursing staff to the need to review control action earlier in the drug treatment process. Sampling technique and equipment would have been examined. Sampling frequency would have been increased to 15-minute intervals.

Control action, including the choice and dose of medication, would have been taken sooner using statistical process control. The prescribed medication, dopamine, a drug which raises blood pressure, would have been identified as a potential cause of the unnecessarily high systolic pressure.

Because medical record data fails to record the sequence and order of data using control charts, the care givers (physicians and nurses) delayed control action which would have improved the quality of patient care. This intensive care patient was at unnecessary risk for a prolonged period of time.

TEACHING EXAMPLE

PAGE 1 OF 5

Clinic	Department Nursing	Chart Individuals
Service Intensive Care Unit	Characteristic Systolic Pressure	Specification $\overline{X}$ = 140 (Desired Mean)
Sample Size ①	Sample Frequency Every Half Hour	Control Limits Calculated By: Date

Average = 174 Upper Control Limit = 198 Lower Control Limit = 150

$\overline{X}$

Average = 9 UCL = 29 LCL = None Moving Ranges

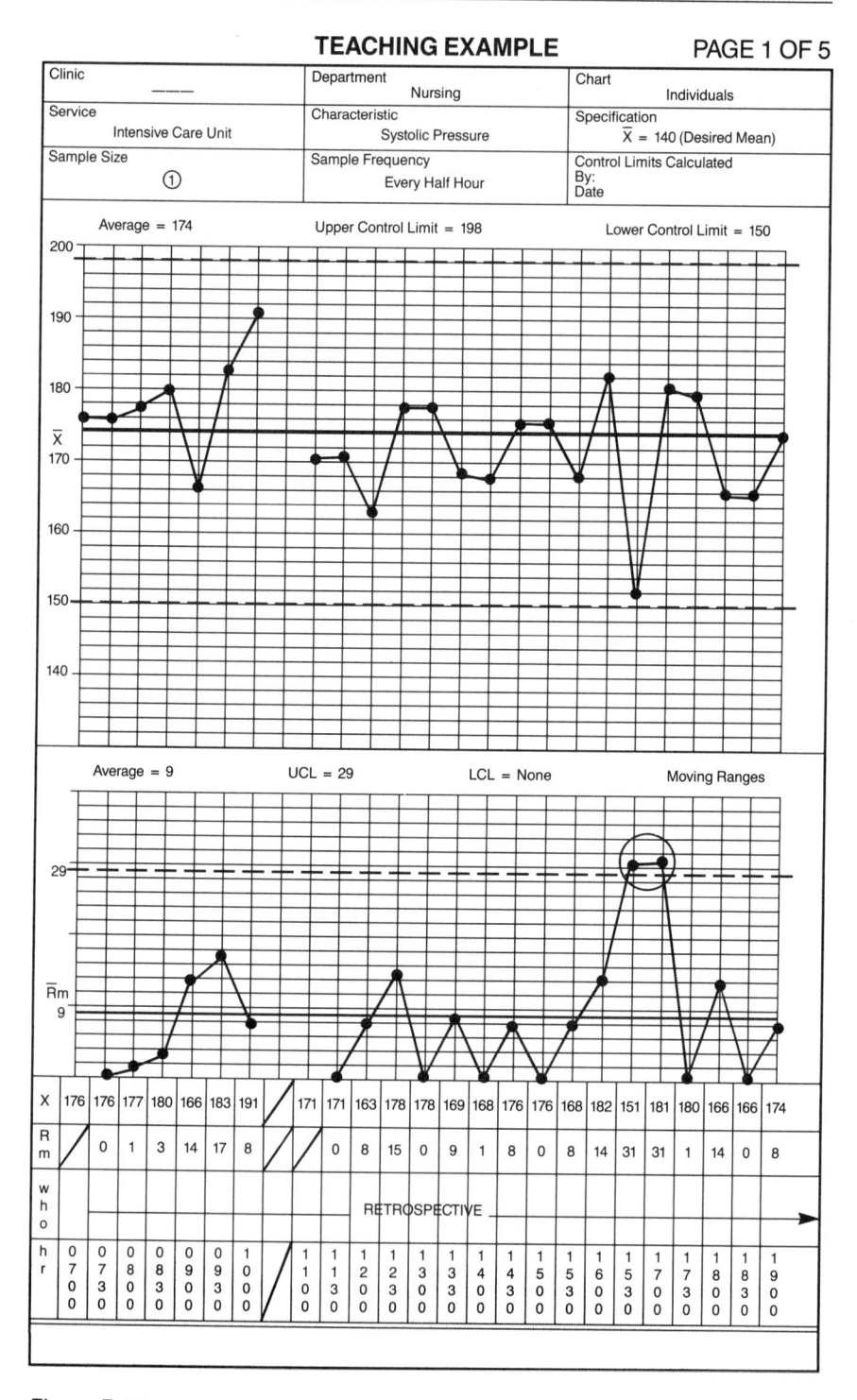

$\overline{Rm}$ = 9

X	176	176	177	180	166	183	191		171	171	163	178	178	169	168	176	168	182	151	181	180	166	166	174
Rm		0	1	3	14	17	8		0	8	15	0	9	1	8	0	8	14	31	31	1	14	0	8
who								RETROSPECTIVE																→
hr	0700	0730	0800	0830	0900	0930	1000		1100	1130	1200	1230	1300	1330	1400	1430	1500	1530	1600	1630	1700	1730	1800	1900

Figure B.4.1

APPENDIX B

TEACHING EXAMPLE   PAGE 2 OF 5

Clinic	Department	Chart
----	Nursing	Individuals
Service	Characteristic	Specification
Intensive Care Unit	Systolic Pressure	$\bar{X}$ = 140 (Desired Mean)
Sample Size	Sample Frequency	Control Limits Calculated
①	Every Half Hour	By: Date ·

Average = 142   Upper Control Limit = 190   Lower Control Limit = 94

Average = 18   UCL = 59   LCL = None   Moving Ranges

X	166	174	166	165	171	162	162	158	111	165	168	153	161	111	133	108	161	117	107	110	106	111	120	151
Rm		8	8	1	6	9	0	4	47	54	3	15	8	50	22	25	53	44	10	7	4	5	9	31

who RETROSPECTIVE →

| hr | 1930 | 2000 | 2030 | 2100 | 2130 | 2200 | 2230 | 2300 | 2330 | 2400 | 0030 | 0100 | 0130 | 0200 | 0230 | 0300 | 0330 | 0400 | 0430 | 0500 | 0530 | 0600 | 0630 | 0700 | 0730 |

Figure B.4.2

TEACHING EXAMPLE   PAGE 3 OF 5

Clinic	Department Nursing	Chart Individuals
Service Intensive Care Unit	Characteristic Diastolic Pressure	Specification $\bar{X}$ = 75 (Desired Mean)
Sample Size ①	Sample Frequency Every Half Hour	Control Limits Calculated By: Date ・

Average = 84   Upper Control Limit = 100   Lower Control Limit = 68

Average = 6   UCL = 20   LCL = None   Moving Ranges

X	61	65	67	77	100	94	92		80	80	93	83	96	91	87	83	86	86	83	88	79	86	91	84	92
Rm		4	2	10	13	6	2		0	13	10	13	5	4	4	3	0	3	5	11	7	5	7	8
who								RETROSPECTIVE																	→
hr	0700	0730	0800	0830	0900	0930	1000	1030	1100	1130	1200	1230	1300	1330	1400	1430	1500	1530	1600	1630	1700	1730	1800	1830	1900

Figure B.4.3

TEACHING EXAMPLE — PAGE 4 OF 5

Clinic	Department: Nursing	Chart: Individuals
Service: Intensive Care Unit	Characteristic: Diastolic Pressure	Specification: $\bar{X}$ = 75 (Desired Mean)
Sample Size: ①	Sample Frequency: Every Half Hour	Control Limits Calculated By: / Date:

Average = 82   Upper Control Limit = 106   Lower Control Limit = 58

Average = 9   UCL = 29   LCL = None   Moving Ranges

X	83	88	85	88	93	86	63	87	88	88	84	75	91	82	89	77	73	84	86	65	62	86		
Rm		5	3	3	5	7	23	24	1	0	4	9	16	9	7	12	4	11	2	21	3	24		
who										RETROSPECTIVE														→
hr	1930	2000	2030	2100	2130	2200	2230	2300	2330	2400	0100	0130	0200	0230	0300	0330	0400	0430	0500	0530	0600	0630		0700

Figure B.4.4

TEACHING EXAMPLE — PAGE 5 OF 5

Clinic	Department	Chart
————	Nursing	Individuals
Service	Characteristic	Specification
Intensive Care Unit	Urine Output	Not Less Than 30cc/Hour
Sample Size	Sample Frequency	Control Limits Calculated
① cc	Hourly	By: Date

Average = 92   Upper Control Limit = 212   Lower Control Limit = 0

$\bar{X}$

Average = 45   UCL = 147   LCL = None   Moving Ranges

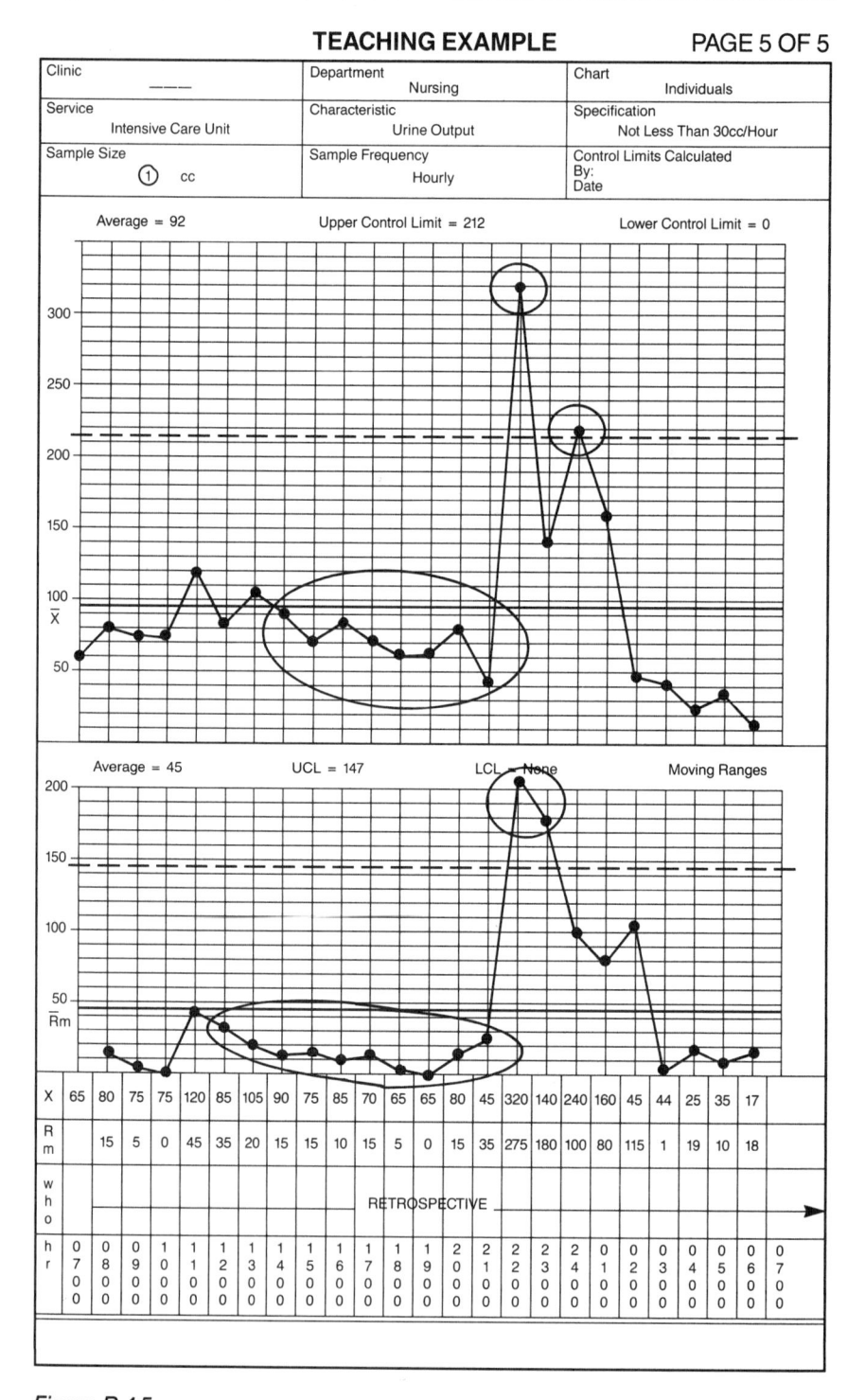

$\bar{R}m$

X	65	80	75	75	120	85	105	90	75	85	70	65	65	80	45	320	140	240	160	45	44	25	35	17
Rm		15	5	0	45	35	20	15	15	10	15	5	0	15	35	275	180	100	80	115	1	19	10	18
who									RETROSPECTIVE															
hr	0700	0800	0900	1000	1100	1200	1300	1400	1500	1600	1700	1800	1900	2000	2100	2200	2300	2400	0100	0200	0300	0400	0500	0600	0700

Figure B.4.5

APPENDIX B

CRITICAL CARE RAW DATA

		0700	0800	0900	1000	1100	1200	1300	1400	1500	1600	1700	1800	1900	2000	2100	2200	2300	2400	0100	0200	0300	0400	0500	0600
Blood Pressure	Hour	176/61	177/67	166/100	191/92	171/80	163/93	178/96	168/87	176/86	182/83	181/79	166/91	174/92	165/88	162/88	158/86	165/87	153/88	111/75	108/82	117/77	110/84	111/65	151/86
	15	167/56	179/75	175/92	206/85												142/90								160/90
	30	176/65	180/77	183/94		171/80	178/83	169/91	176/83	168/86	151/88	180/86	166/84	166/83	171/85	162/93	111/63	168/88	161/84	133/91	161/89	107/73	106/86	120/62	
	45	162/74	181/82	191/86		171/105											84/69		110/71		105/68			121/92	135/82
Output		0700	0800	0900	1000	1100	1200	1300	1400	1500	1600	1700	1800	1900	2000	2100	2200	2300	2400	0100	0200	0300	0400	0500	0600
Urine		65	80	75	75	120	85	105	90	75	85	70	65	65	80	45	320	140	240	160	45	44	25	35	17

Figure B.5.1 Variable data collected in time ordered sequence.

Conclusion

Doctors want to treat depression, tobacco abuse, alcohol abuse, and inactivity. They want to improve dietary habits. But, they do not have the statistical tools, the training, or the time to do so effectively.

They use their memory for complex clinical decisions instead of using flow diagrammed quality protocols. They use opinion to monitor treatment outputs instead of statistical process control.

Quality health care insists on prevention, accurate diagnosis, and treatment plans which mandate teamwork. Statistical method from the viewpoint of quality control gives the team the power to monitor, control, and improve process outputs.

Chronic diseases like diabetes and high blood pressure can be eliminated as outputs. When they cannot be eliminated the effects of these diseases can be minimized through process quality control.

Flow diagrammed quality protocols minimize reliance on physician memory. In this case study a completely different medication from what the patient had been taking would have been prescribed. There are several pharmacologic reasons for this.

Thiazide-type diuretics like chlorthalidone have metabolic effects that increase coronary risk. These drugs adversely affect the lipid profile, raising triglyceride and low-density lipoprotein levels. Diuretics also slightly increase the serum glucose level, possibly exacerbating glucose intolerance in diabetics. Diuretics lower serum potassium which may increase the risk of dangerous and fatal arrhythmias.

The cause of death in the case study was cardiac arrhythmia. Cardiac arrhythmia may have been caused by the patient's prescribed medicine.

(In our teaching example the medication dose would have been adjusted more quickly, saving money, and improving care.)

Beta-blockers also adversely affect lipid profiles. They interfere with exercise tolerance. They decrease renal perfusion by decreasing cardiac output, possibly further compromising renal function in diabetics. Plus, beta-blockers interfere with the body's response to insulin-induced hypoglycemia, masking the warning signs of impending insulin shock.[9] They cause depression, and impotence.

ACE inhibitors and calcium channel blockers, on the other hand, do not have adverse metabolic effects. They may even improve the lipid profile and cause regression of left ventricular hypertrophy.[4] ACE inhibitors may improve or stabilize renal function in diabetics.[9] However, serum K+ and creatinine must be monitored closely in a patient with diabetes when beginning therapy with an ACE inhibitor. Chronic cough is a side effect in 3 percent of patients.

Flow diagrams improve health care quality by decreasing variation. They add consistency, discipline, and thoroughness. Statistical process control adds precision and accuracy to any treatment protocol, including drug therapy.

Processes produce outputs. Process outputs can be controlled. Outputs can be predictable within the limits of probability.

Health, not disease, can become the manufactured product.

INDEX

A
Accidental injuries, 8
ACE inhibitors, 186
Act, in integrated teamwork, 96
Acute alcohol toxicity, 8
Addiction, 9
Administrator, 40-42
Aetna's Federal Employees' Health Benefits Program, 97
AIDS risk, 44
Alcohol abuse, 6, 7, 8
  employment screening policy for, 122-23
Alcohol dependence syndrome, 8
Alcohol polyneuropathy, 8
Alcohol psychosis, 8
Alcoholic cardiomyopathy, 8
Alcoholic gastritis, 8
Alcoholics Anonymous, 103
Alcohol-related debilitation, 8
A priori assumption, 23-24, 81
  definition of, 23
  in traditional medical model, 24
Average, 26

B
Beck Depression Inventory, 108, 111, 172
Behavioral medicine, 127
Behavioral science, 132, 133
Bell-shaped curve, 27

Beta-blockers, 186
Bladder cancer, 7
Blood cholesterol, 7
Blue Cross/Blue Shield, 41, 97
Brainpower, characteristics of, 104
Brief therapy, 97-101, 133

C
Calcium channel blockers, 186
Cancer, 7
   cost of care for terminally
     ill, 11
"Captain of the ship" doctrine, 81
Cardiovascular disease, 7
Carter Center Study, 5-6, 86, 91
Case mix management, 82
Catastrophic disease, 7
Cause-and-effect diagrams, 105
Center for Disease Control's
  computerized health risk
  appraisal, 172
Chance life stressors, 123
Change, and medical science, xi
Chaos, 29
Charts, importance of, 55, 59, 60
Check, in integrated
  teamwork, 96
Check sheets, 104, 105
Chronic diseases, 186
Circular logic, 77
Cirrhosis, 8
Clark, Barney, 5
*Closing the Gap, The Burden of
Unnecessary Illness*, 5-6
Cocaine intoxication, 8
Conceptual pragmatism, 22, 24
Congressional initiative, 131-34
Consumer, role of, in World Class
  Health Care, 118-19
Control chart formulas, 29
Control charts, 24-25, 25, 30, 76, 105, 106-7
Cost shifting, 42
Costs of quality health care
  accounting system, 128
    appraisal investments, 129
    external failures, 129, 131

    internal failures, 129
    prevention investments, 128-29
Craniotomy, 40
Crisis management, 32
Cynicism, 12-15

D
Daily rounds, case history of, 66-68
Data order sequence, 29
Data sequence, importance of
  original, 20-21
Deductive thought, 21, 22
Deming, W. Edwards, 21, 32, 120-21, 125, 132
Deming cycle, 21
  versus Shewhart cycle, 22
Depression, costs of, 10
DeShazer, Steve, 98
Diabetes, 171
*Diagnostic and Statistical Manual
3rd Edition Revised (DSM-III-R)*, 38, 82
Diagnostic protocols in world
  class health care, 87
Diagnostic Related Groups
  (DRGs), 40, 81-82
Diet, 7
Disease process, 76
  genesis of, 24
Diuretics, 186
Do, in integrated teamwork, 95
Drug abuse, employment
  screening policy for, 122-23

E
Education, 132
  in health care system, 117-18
  in integrated treatment, 101-4
Effect, law of, 91
80/20 rule. *See* Pareto principle.
Einstein, Albert, 22, 23, 24, 73, 75
Empiricism, 22
Employee assistance program
  (EAP), 129
    establishment of, 123

Employer initiative, 120-25
Employment screening policy,
    establishment of, 122-23
End of life expenses, 11-12
Epistemology, 22

F
Family initiative, 119-20
Federal government, restricting
    access to care by, xii
Fiduciary responsibility, 41
Fishbone diagram, 105
Flow diagrams, 105, 169
    in quality protocols, 186
Formal distribution theory, 25
Frequency, law of, 91
Frequency interval, 101-2
Frequency ratio, 101
Fuchs, Victor, xi

G
Gamblers Anonymous, 103
Gingrich, Rosanne D., 169
Goal, in integrated teamwork,
    93, 95

H
Habitual behavior, 9
Health care
    construction, 40
    managing the change to
        quality, 81-84
    quality approach to, 31
    teamwork in, 31-32
Health care costs, xii, 5, 38
Health care model, cynicism in,
    12-15
Health care payment system, 9-10
Health care supplier certification
    process
    establishment of, 124-25
    sample program, 149-67
Health care system
    access to, xii
    cynicism, 12-15
    delivery of, 19
    end of life expenses, 11-12

misbehavior in, 7
    accidents, 8
    cancer, 7
    cardiovascular disease, 7
    cirrhosis, 8
    homicide, 8-10
    suicide, 8-10
    problems associated with, 5-6
    psychological distress, 10-11
Health habits, 116
Health insurance, lack of, 9
Health problems, diagnosis of, 10
Health promotion, 42
Histograms, 26, 104, 105
Holmes and Rahe Social
    Readjustment Rating Scale, 172
Homicide, 8-10
Hospital administrators, 36
Hospital bill, size of average, 9
Hospitalization, as a teachable
    moment, 91-92
Hypertension, 171
    quality protocol for, 172-78

I
Individual initiative, 116-19
Inductive reasoning, 21, 22,
    25, 31
Insurance, 126-27
INSURE project, 103-4
Integrated treatment, 92
    education, 101-4
    medical cost offset effect,
        96-101
    plan, do, check, act, 93-96
    process quality control, 104-111
Intensive care unit, case study in,
    68-69
International Classification of
Diseases, 9th Revision, Clinical
Modification (ICD-9-CM), 38, 82
Intuition, 22
Ishikawa, 125
Ishikawa diagram, 105

J
Johnson, Lyndon B., 40

Juran, J. M., 125, 128, 132

K
Kaiser Permanente, 96-97
Kaizen principle, 79-81, 133
Knowledge
   as probable only, 23
   components of, 77-78
   importance of mathematics
     to, 25
Kuhn, Thomas, 73, 133

L
Laryngeal cancer, 7
Lewis, C. I., 22, 23, 25, 73,
   75-77, 108
Lifestyle rewards, 9
Lung cancer, 7

M
Malpractice cases
   possibility of, 92
   and World Class Health
     Care, 116
Mass inspection approach to
   quality control, xii
Mathematical proof, 31
Mathematical statistics, 132
Mathematics, importance of, to
   knowledge, 25
Median, 26
Medicaid, 9, 41
Medical cost containment, xi
Medical cost offset effect,
   96-101, 133
Medical marketing, 13
Medical process outputs,
   inspection of, 12-13
Medical protocols, 12
Medical records, 69-70, 104-5
Medical science, 13, 127-28, 132
   and change, xi
Medical technology, as tool, xi-xii
Medical tradition
   a priori assumption in, 24
   versus World Class Health
     Care, 169-87

Medicare, 9, 41
Medicine, stages of, 74
Michigan Alcoholism Screening
   Test, 108, 110, 172
Misbehavior
   accidental injuries, 8
   cancer, 7
   cardiovascular disease, 7
   cirrhosis, 8
   homicide, 8
   suicide, 8-10
Mode, 26
Monopsony, 131
Mothers Against Drunk Drivers
   (MADD), 119
Multidisciplinary approach to
   treatment, 24

N
Natural law of large numbers, 30
Nurse educator, in integrated
   treatment, 92, 96

O
Obstetrical services, 41
Overcontrol, 29
Overeaters Anonymous, 103

P
Pancreatic cancer, 7
Pareto, Vilfredo, 6
Pareto analysis, 174
Pareto charts, 104-05, 105
Pareto principle, 6, 95
Patient, 36
   in integrated treatment, 92,
     93-95, 96
Patient-doctor relation, cynicism
   in, 12
Patient education, 38
P chart, 123
Physician, 36, 37-39
   in health care system, 117
   in integrated treatment, 92, 96
Plan, in integrated teamwork,
   93-96
Pneumonia, 8

Policies, 125-26
Pre-employment screening policy, 123
Prevention investments, 128-29
Prevention services, lack of, 7
Primary prevention, 6
　gaps in, 6
Problem resolution in World Class Health Care, 87-89
Process output, 171
Process quality control, 104-111
　statistical tools of, 17
Psychiatric care unit, 70-72
Psychological assessment, need for comprehensive, 120
Psychological distress, 10-11
Psychologist, in integrated treatment, 92, 96
Psychotherapeutic support, 10
Psychotherapy, 98

Q
Quality approach to health care, 31
Quality control, mass inspection approach to, xii
Quality health care protocols
　characteristics of, 171
　flow diagrammed, 186
　for hypertension, 172-78
Quality improvement, 150
Quality initiatives, 115-16
　congressional initiative, 131-34
　employer initiative, 120-25
　　adopt a World Class Health Care philosophy, 121
　　build a consensus for quality, 121-22
　　costs of quality health care accounting system, 128-31
　　establish a health care supplier certification process, 124-28
　　establish an employee assistance program, 123
　　establish an employment screening policy, 122-23
　　negotiate for quality, with service and coverage, 123-24
　family initiative, 119-20
　individual initiative, 116-19
Quality report, goals of, 108
Quill, T. E., 10

R
Readiness, law of, 91
Relative Value System (RVS), 38, 82, 89-90, 133
Resource-Based Relative Value Scale, 89-90
Run charts, 105

S
Scatter diagrams, 107
Scattergrams, 105
Scientific discipline, stages of, 74
Scientific revolution, 74-75
Second opinions, 82
Self-help groups, 103
Shewhart, Walter A., xii, 20, 21, 22, 23, 24, 25, 26, 29, 30, 74, 75, 77-78, 108, 125, 132
Shewhart cycle, 21
　versus Deming cycle, 22
Shewhart-Deming cycle, 77, 92-96
　circular logic of, 96
Smoking, 7
Somatization, 10-11
State government, restricting access to care by, xii
Statistical control, 29
Statistical process control (SPC), 22, 24, 30-31, 132
　as philosophy, 152
　primary steps to, 20
Statistical process control charts, 169
Statistical reasoning, 24, 75
Statistical thinking, 96
StorageTek Process Quality Rating Program, 150
Suicide, 8-10
Supplier certification programs
　establishment of, 124-25

process quality rating (PQR), 150-67
sample, 149-67
Surgeon General, 91
Symptoms, 12

T
Tampering, xii, 24, 29, 31
Tavistock Institute, 127
Teamwork
    in health care, 31-32
    in integrated treatment, 92
    in World Class Health Care, 86-87, 125
Therapy flow diagram, 98
Therapy role play, 71
Thiazide-type diuretics, 186
Thorndike, Edward L., 91
Tobacco, 7
Trauma care, case histories in, 43-59
Trist, Eric, 115, 127
Tuberculosis, 8

U
Undercontrol, 29
Utilization review, 81, 82

W
Weight Watchers, 103
Wells, H. G., 96
World Class Health Care, 32, 73-84
    access to care in, 115-16
    adopting philosophy for, 121
    and behavioral medicine, 127
    cost-effective treatment in, 89-90
    diagnostic protocols in, 87
    hospitalization as teachable moment, 91-92
    insurance, 126-27
    integrated treatment in, 92
        act, 96
        check, 96
        do, 95
        education, 101-4
        medical cost offset effect, 96-101
        plan, 93-96
        process quality control, 104-11
    Kaizen principle in, 79-81
    Lewis's theory of knowledge, 75-77
    and malpractice cases, 116
    managing change to quality health care, 81-84
    market demand for, 78-79
    and medical science, 127-28
    versus medical tradition, 169-87
    negotiations in, 123-24
    policies in, 125-26
    pragmatic approach of, 75
    problem resolution in, 87-89
    scientific approach in, 76-77
    Shewhart's components of knowledge in, 77-78
    teamwork in, 86-87, 125
World Class Health Care insurers, 126-27
World Class Health Care Process, 84-91
World Class Health Care value payment system, 133